The Sex Myth

Why everything we're told is wrong

Dr Brooke Magnanti

WEIDENFELD & NICOLSON

LONDON

First published in Great Britain in 2012 by Weidenfeld & Nicolson
An imprint of the Orion Publishing Group Ltd
Orion House, 5 Upper St Martin's Lane
London WC2H 9EA

An Hachette UK Company

(Trade paperback) 978 0 2978 6639 8
(Ebook) 978 0 2978 6640 4

A CIP catalogue record for this book is
available from the British Library.

Typeset by Input Data Services Ltd, Bridgwater, Somerset

Printed and bound by CPI Group (UK) Ltd, Croydon, CR0 4YY

www.orionbooks.co.uk

Contents

Introduction

Men, it has been well said, think in herds; it will be seen that they go mad in herds, while they only recover their senses slowly, and one by one.

Charles Mackay,
Extraordinary Popular Delusions and the Madness of Crowds

Sex is virtually a human universal. It's something most of us can claim, if not expertise, at least an enthusiastic amateur interest.

Plenty of people have opinions about sex, sex work, and sexuality, and why not? When it comes to something of which we have (ahem) hands-on experience, we can all be experts. But sex is a broad topic, the inner workings of which are still somewhat of a mystery to us, no matter how much we practise. Once out of the comfort zone of what we know first hand, all kinds of strange rumours can take hold. And once a rumour starts to spread it can be very hard to stop.

Relying on others for our information about sex and sexuality starts young. I had an early personal lesson in how curiosity and lack of information mix.

When I was eight years old, kids in my year spent a lot of time trying to catch a glimpse of the opposite sex in the nude. The boys may have started it, but we girls were good at outsmarting them.

By the time the summer break came the challenge was at fever pitch. We lived in a small town by the beach and most of us went to the same places together, chaperoned by parents and relatives. A lucky few had older brothers and sisters with cars. The beach turned out to be the perfect place to spy. For one thing the doors of the changing rooms ended a crucial several inches above the ground. In the minds of the girls it was therefore theoretically possible, if we were quiet enough, to win this little war.

Because I was the youngest and smallest in the group (a good three years younger than those in the same class at school, and shorter than average with it), the job of official eye was given to me. What I quickly discovered was that the couple of inches between the floor and the bottom of the changing-room doors didn't allow me to see anything of interest. The angles were all wrong. At most I might glimpse a part of someone's foot, but only if they were standing close to the gap. Otherwise all I could see was the tiled floor of the boys' changing area.

Weeks passed and the speculation about what the boys were hiding grew more elaborate. Clearly we were just as motivated as they were to find out what the opposite sex was up to, but who knew how it would end?

One morning a girl called Tanya finished the war for good. She said there was a hole in the door of the boys' changing room and she had seen what they looked like naked. We gathered round, ready to receive all the gory details. But as for secondary sources, well, those didn't exist. We would have to take her word for it.

According to Tanya, the male member was long, with a spiral ridge running down it – a lot like a screw, in fact. Curiously satisfied by this explanation, we forgot about the challenge and went back to enjoying the beach for the rest of the summer. We could now all say with confidence what boys looked like naked without having to actually, you know, see one. No one gave the details of the story a second thought even though they didn't make much sense. After all, if there was a hole in the door of the changing room, why did no one else know about it? Wouldn't the boys have realised someone was spying on them? Wasn't it odd that the shape she described – a screw – just happened to coincide with a popular euphemism for having sex?

As the teenage years progressed, similar gossip fires raged through school every year. The stories passed between girls became more sophisticated and corrected a lot of the faults in Tanya's information. But we weren't only interested in naked people any more. The gossip was more often about who was doing what with whom. And, of course, the juicy parts always happened at times and in places where no one could prove otherwise. There was a notebook reserved especially for recording our gossip and speculations. It was passed around during French and RE. We didn't question the authority of the notebook. If it was written, it was true, no matter how unlikely the event – or whose reputation was smashed because of it. We were at the age when we couldn't get enough of thinking and talking about sex.

From the first rumours in the schoolyard to the first fumblings in the dark, has there ever been a topic more talked about, thought about, and argued about? We begin to learn about sex and sexuality from the things we tell each other, and later from our own experiences.

As we get older and gain more insight, our gaze widens: from *when will I have sex? What will it be like? How are other people doing it?* to broader questions of sexual orientation, relationships, and gender issues. We're fascinated with the periphery of sex as well as the nuts and bolts of it. Stories about prostitution, porn, and sex crimes are guaranteed to get news coverage, magazine features, and column inches in the papers. Memoirs, exposés, and kiss-and-tells fly off the shelves. We get our expertise however we can.

But the less direct experience we have, the more we turn back to gathering knowledge the old-fashioned way. The schoolyard way. 'I know someone who knows someone ...' once again becomes a believable source of information.

For example, it was once easy for people to believe second-hand stories and rumours about homosexuality, because most people didn't know anyone who was out. As homosexuality became more open and more visible, and therefore more people knew that they knew gay people, the malicious rumours and hatred began to wane. According to polls by the *Washington Post* and ABC News, the percentage of people supporting equal marriage rights for gay couples has risen in direct proportion with the acceptance and visibility of gay people. Nasty prejudices and damaging assumptions have been vanquished by the plain light of day.

Other groups, however, who are not yet as accepted can still experience the full brunt of the rumour mill's attacks. Because a lot of us don't personally know anyone in sex work, old stereotypes continue to hold sway in that area. Without direct knowledge, who's to say otherwise? Who dares put their hand up first to challenge what most people believe to be true?

What is clear is that we need some way of telling what is real from what is myth.

Luckily, there is just such an approach that can help sort the truth from the fiction. The methods of scientific inquiry, which describe researchers' discoveries about the physical world, are a useful template for finding out what is true and what is false in the realm of human society and sexuality.

While sexual manuals like the *Kama Sutra* have existed for centuries, the systematic study of human sexuality really started in the late nineteenth century with Krafft-Ebing's *Psychopathia Sexualis* and has only been a cohesive academic discipline since the mid-twentieth century.

Many early works in what is sometimes called 'sexology' reflected not only the fruits of scientific inquiry, but also the morality of their time. For instance, Krafft-Ebing believed procreation to be the only legitimate purpose for sex, so any sex activity not resulting in pregnancy was a 'perversion'. He considered rape to be 'aberrant' but not a perversion – since it is possible for rape to result in pregnancy. It's an interpretation that would be absolutely scandalous for a scientist to hold now.

Just as our attitudes change, so too do the tools of research and analysis. These changes can complement each other in unexpected and beneficial ways. Now the focus on what is testable and verifiable has taken root in the study of sex and gender, there is less acceptance of personal opinion as the only source of evidence.

This, by the way, is a good thing. The results of the new generation of studies can be controversial, because they have the power to contradict our assumptions. But challenges are good: being able to re-examine what we think to be the truth is one of the hallmarks of good science and of human achievement.

In recent years a large number of researchers have looked into areas of human experience previously assumed to be untestable. Questions such as whether porn is harmful, or how childhood is affected by sexuality, can now be examined in a way that is consistent with evidence-based reasoning. Not only that, people who study different disciplines are starting to realise the advantages of interdisciplinary study, with social science enriching the finds of quantitative methods and vice versa.

Researchers also share the methods and results of their research, which allows others around the world to test the theories to see if they hold true there too. With the entire research community looking on, it becomes harder and harder to pass off opinion and unverifiable stories as proof. With everyone from governments to parents concerned about sex and sexuality, a solid base should emerge on which to build public policy and law.

Using these approaches, we can now begin to know the truth about humans, gender, and sex. Some of the findings have been consistent with things that we already thought were true but, as with Galileo's rejection of the flat Earth, sometimes the evidence shows a completely different reality. Sometimes challenging the status quo attracts controversy.

Why? Partly because so much of our lives depends not on studies, but on conforming to the mores and opinions of our social group. Media plays a role in this, with everything from news to sitcoms reinforcing stereotypes about sex and relationships. With so much invested in a particular way of seeing the world it can be easy to write off the truth as something we don't, or can't, know.

And there is a lot of energy invested in maintaining the status quo. For every study demonstrating that our preconceived ideas about sex might be wrong, there is someone ready to derail the logical argument by claiming they know better. For every statistic that is produced by intellectually honest researchers, there is a manipulated or exaggerated guess being promoted by someone with a hidden agenda.

Back in the fifth century BC, ancient Greek philosophy was

surrounded by similar controversy. On one side were the sophists, among them Gorgias, who persuaded the public to ignore experts and listen to him instead, and Protagoras, who advocated making the worst case in an argument appear stronger. For a while, they were influential and successful. Their techniques were sought out by noblemen going after public office. Whether they knew about a topic or not, the sophists were very good at using language to impress an audience. They formed their arguments regardless of the relevant facts. The sophists charged high fees to their students, while other teachers such as Socrates charged nothing. The sophists attacked Socrates and Plato for questioning them and their methods of misinformation. In the end, truth won out over the sophists' quest for money and power. But it's a battle that is fought endlessly.

AIDS denialism and anti-evolution movements are just a couple of examples where emotional arguments sometimes gain the upper hand over evidence and reason. The MMR debate was problematic as well. The viewpoints promoted by these arguments may seem laughable to some, but their proponents have been skilled at introducing doubt, and therefore influencing the general public.

Aristotle said that truths have 'a natural tendency to prevail over their opposites', but with so much misinformation saturating the media, it takes time and effort. Researchers are often deeply buried in their disciplines. They do not always have the resources to ensure their work is being represented accurately. This leaves the door open to those with other agendas who can then twist and manipulate the facts. In situations where logic should rule, it is catchphrases, high emotions, and prejudice that take control.

But there is a growing hunger for the truth. More and more people are questioning whether what they see in the papers is reality, and whether the gut feelings they've been told to give way to are real. Look behind the numbers reported in the media and you'll see what they really mean. Dig that bit deeper below the surface and you'll discover more information than ever before. What you thought you knew often turns out to be what you didn't know at all.

This book will be looking at some of the most persistent myths about sex and sexuality, and examining the evidence that supports and rejects the stories we hear every day. It's a step up from trying to peek under the changing-room door – and hopefully a lot more illuminating.

1

MYTH: When it comes to sexual attraction, men are visually stimulated and always interested in sex – and women aren't.

The great question that has never been answered, and which I have not yet been able to answer, despite my thirty years of research into the feminine soul, is "What does a woman want?"

Sigmund Freud, 1907

Sex is everywhere. Sex sells. Sex is a biological urge, a natural part of life, and the most fun you can have without laughing – though it's even better if you do. Sex is a beautiful thing between two people ... and between five it's fantastic.

Or is it? For as many times as sex is painted as a natural, enjoyable activity, it's also portrayed as something women use to get things from men, or put up with in a relationship, or don't really enjoy. Over and again men are stereotyped as slaves to their desires – and women are stereotyped as disinterested schemers who only use their erotic powers as a path to domestic bliss.

Porn and erotic entertainment are presumed to appeal only to men, and women just want the relationship. Even in homosexual relationships it's assumed gay men are all into anonymous sex, and gay women just want to build nests together. It's a broad generalisation, and not even really true. So, where on earth has this myth come from?

Consider the output of the amusingly named Cambridge Women's Pornography Cooperative. Their work, including the book *Porn for Women*, largely consists of images of fully clothed men dusting, washing dishes, and tidying up. Why? Because, according to the publisher's blurb, 'A world where clothes get folded just so, delicious dinners await, and flatulence is just not that funny ... is porn that will leave women begging for more!' While a certain amount of the book is no doubt ironic, it also says a lot about widespread assumptions regarding women and sex. In other words, women couldn't possibly be turned on by images of sex, and what they really want is ... a man maid.

Of course, women wouldn't actually be turned on by something as simplistic as an image of an excited naked man ... or would they? We're used to thinking of men as being the visual ones. Women's sexual response is a function not of physical lust but of emotional arousal, right?

When it comes to what triggers lust, there are some things you hear over and over: men are visually stimulated, women aren't. Men will chase anyone, women are more discriminating.

The majority of pornography consumers are men, and so are the customers of strip clubs. Male clients of prostitutes far outnumber female clients. There is no equivalent to lads' magazines like *Nuts* and *Zoo* marketed for women, and most attempts to emulate such things have failed utterly. Page Seven Fellas, the *Sun's* beefcake counterpart to their topless Page Three Girls, was distinctly short-lived.

The idea that male sexuality is predominantly visual while women's is not is taken as self-evident.

Hence the Cambridge Women's Pornography Cooperative, with their soft-focus images of stereotypically handsome men lighting candles and drawing the bath being presented as 'porn that will leave women begging for more'. Women's desire has been ceded as a territory so unknown it is presumed to exist only in the mind, and only in a state of emotional contentment. So, instead of hot scenes of sex, women get domestic chores being served up as a suitable substitute for the naked body. And women who are always 'up for it'? As rare as unicorns.

But while the popular assumption is that female desire is something unknowable, alchemical, difficult to pin down ... increasing volumes of research in human sexuality are showing otherwise.

At Northwestern University in Illinois, J Michael Bailey and his research colleagues conduct experiments into the practicalities of arousal. Traditional research hands out questionnaires about romantic and sexual preferences and that's all. Bailey's group doesn't just rely on people self-reporting their sexual likes and dislikes – it also measures genital response. After all, what someone says they like can be influenced by any number of factors: discomfort with admitting to being turned on, or a desire to be seen as 'normal'. Our disinclination to be perfectly honest when discussing sex is high. Even in the laboratory setting and even when anonymity is assured.

It's their results with women that are especially interesting. The difference between what women report is turning them on and what is actually getting their bodies to respond, is significant. We may think we know what turns people on, but the data are giving researchers a very different picture.

Previous studies of men and sexual orientation showed that, in general, male responses are straightforward. Heterosexual men respond strongly to heterosexual porn, and weakly to homosexual porn. For gay men, it's the opposite: gay porn turns them on; the hetero stuff, not so much. So, for men, the psychological and physiological desires are in sync – what turns them on is also what they report enjoying emotionally.

This is so reliable in men, in fact, that detecting physical arousal has even been used to accurately identify men who are 'still in the closet' – the ones who have homosexual desires but are not yet willing to admit to them.

This pattern of male physical response could be partly to do with the obviousness of their arousal. Men get erections. It's clear to other people. But, more importantly, it's clear to the men. There is a direct, observable connection between a man's physical response and his level of sexual interest. Associating the two in his mind? It's easy. It's also undeniable.

The assumption that women lack interest in sex may start, partly, with anatomical differences. When we look at male and female bodies, there are obvious differences. Men, with outwardly placed genitalia, come with an external signal of when they're turned on. You know it. They know it. The whole world knows it. Women, on the other hand, don't come with such an obvious sign. Male desire is apparent, whereas for reasons as much to do with cultural norms as biology, both sexes can be unclear about a woman's sexual signals.

This is something of a double-edged sword. It isn't always apparent when women are turned on, so you could assume they aren't. On the other hand, the ambiguity does perhaps give women the upper hand as *providers* of eroticism.

Consider strippers, for instance. Why is it that female strippers are far more successful than their male counterparts? There are far more women in stripping than there are men, and the women can earn much more. The usual assumption is that this is because men have stronger libidos and a greater desire to see the opposite sex naked. But could it be something else entirely? After all, a woman taking off her clothes for the entertainment of men is erotically ambiguous. She could theoretically be aroused, and the arousal of others is, in its turn, arousing to the viewer. In other words, women are able to fake it.

A man stripping for the enjoyment of women, however, is less ambiguous. It is obvious even before the quick-release hot pants come off whether a male stripper is actually turned on by the situation he's in. If he isn't erect – and male strippers generally aren't – he is as sexless as a Ken doll. The signals of the potential partner being turned on, and thus turning on the viewer, are all but absent. Hard abs are simply no substitute.

This difference between signs of men's and women's arousal may also affect porn. Women are the high earners, and their orgasmic performances may or may not be genuine. Men, on the other hand, are paid a lot less, and the pressure to deliver the authentic goods? Pretty high. The same goes for prostitution: women can fake it until the client makes it – guys can't. And in the high end of sex work, a call girl will have more work and higher pay than her male counterparts.

So, it seems that at least part of the assumption that women don't really enjoy sex is based on the observation that they don't necessarily have to be in the mood to have it. In other words, it may be a stereotype based on the possibility that someone *could* be lying, on feeling potentially insecure about how interested the other party is.

Until recently, the studies matching physical arousal to reported sexual preferences were not done on women. The assumption was that for women, as for men, what they said they enjoyed was exactly the same as what their bodies responded to. But without the corresponding data on physical arousal, there was no actual way of knowing. 'Women's sexuality has been far more neglected than men's in scientific research,' Bailey has said.[1] And when women were examined, the difference in the results was startling.

One of the experiments conducted by Bailey and his colleagues at Northwestern recruited people with strong preferences for a particular sex of partner. In other words, the study included heterosexuals and homosexuals, but not bisexuals. The subjects were presented with films depicting male-male, female-female, and male-female scenes of oral and penetrative sex. The subjects submitted both to objective measurement of genital arousal as well as self-reporting their responses for comparison.[2]

Participants ranked the films in order of how aroused they felt watching them. The heterosexual women in the study ranked male-male films the lowest, followed by female-female in the middle, and finally female-male films the highest. But when the genital arousal data were compared to these rankings, something interesting emerged.

It turned out that the genital engorgement data told a completely different story from what straight women were putting on paper. They claimed male-male porn interested them the least, but looking at the physical response, male-male and female-female films ranked similarly – and very high. On paper, straight women ranked heterosexual pairings as the most arousing ... but their physical response while watching these films was actually *lower* than with the other types of films. Straight women were getting more physically turned on watching homosexual pairings, even films with no women in them at all, than they were by straight scenes. By contrast, over 90 per cent of men showed higher genital arousal for the films that corresponded to their preferred partnerships.

Challenging preconceptions is a huge task, and results that contradict the prevailing assumptions rarely get media coverage. So, while you hear all the time that men and women are turned on by different things, what you rarely hear is that women respond to visual stimuli too.

Researchers at Washington University School of Medicine in St Louis measured the brainwave activity of 264 women viewing a series of slides. The pictures contained various scenes from water skiers to snarling dogs to undressed couples in sensual poses. What did they find? That when the women viewed erotic pictures, their brains produced electrical responses that were stronger than when looking at the other pictures. This difference in brainwave response emerged very quickly, suggesting different neural circuits are involved in processing erotic images.[3] Women, in other words, are susceptible to the visual. It's not only men.

Repeated studies by other research groups support these conclusions. Studies also show that women are consistently physically turned on by gay porn even when they're not gay, and that they're turned on by hetero porn too. They also respond to footage of some of our closest animal relatives, bonobos, mating. And interestingly, even when they identify themselves as heterosexual, women's physiological response to images of sex is wide-ranging. It's not category specific like men's.[4]

Why are these results so different from popular assumptions about women? 'I think that the earlier impression was probably formulated from intuition. You would expect that somebody would show the greatest amount of physical responding to the things that correspond with what they say they like,' said scientist Meredith Chivers, commenting publically on the work. And since previously only men had been tested, there was no data that challenged the assumption. It certainly throws a spanner into the belief that most women don't like or even respond to porn and other erotic imagery.

Dr Chivers, who began her career in Bailey's research group at Northwestern, is particularly interested in the mysteries of female sexual arousal. She agrees that the research about men's preferences matching their physical responses was erroneously applied to women in the past: 'I think that those [male] findings were then extended to women, but the research I've done has shown that model of sexual interest and sexual response doesn't work for women.'

Data showing the reality to be somewhat different from the myth is also backed up by other kinds of studies. Until recently, it was a lot harder to get your hands on erotic images without going into licensed adult shops to buy it. These shops were perceived as unwelcoming and unfriendly to women, and had a mostly deserved reputation for being unsavoury places. Things began to change with the expansion of Ann

Summers, which had originally been a chain of more traditional sex shops. The company started the trend in the 1980s for women-only home parties, where women could buy sex toys and other adult materials surrounded by their close friends and in familiar spaces.

The Ann Summers strategy of making the experience a familiar and comfortable one worked for them on the high street as well, as their chain expanded into 139 brightly lit, female-friendly stores in the UK.[5] Other 'adult superstores' and similar businesses soon followed. Suddenly, buying porn, sexy toys, and racy lingerie was seen as something women could do without undue embarrassment or being perved on by creeps.

But it's actually the availability of sex toys, porn, and other adult services on the internet that has been the greatest equaliser. How do we know? Because of internet search engines, like Google. Search engines record the patterns of what their users look for, with very good cross-referenced information about the age and sex of the people using their services. With Google making their results available to search, some surprising patterns in what men and women are looking at start to emerge.

Google search statistics for 2006 show that terms such as 'porn', 'free porn', and 'playboy' are more likely to be entered by men than by women (96 per cent, 97 per cent, and 86 per cent male users, respectively). So far, so stereotype. Men outnumber women, but only slightly, for searches of 'adult DVD', 'XXX videos', and 'sex toys'. The search terms 'sex', 'sex chat', and 'sexy'? Interestingly, those ones are equally as likely to be entered by women as they are by men. But then the surprise – women are *more* likely to type the search terms 'adult sex', 'free sex', and 'cyber sex' into the search engine than men are.[6]

In the privacy of one's home, at the computer, even what little stigma might arise from wandering into a friendly mainstream shop like Ann Summers is non-existent. It would seem that, once free of the worry of who might see them doing it, women are indeed interested in sex and erotica.

SEX! Now that I have your attention ...

When I was at university, this was by far the most popular advertising ruse for the thousands of fliers littering campus. Whether advertising for a housemate or an upcoming event, *SEX!* was emblazoned on notices posted all over the place – even ones in the women-only dorms. A few wags tried *PIZZA!* for a couple of weeks as an alternative attention-getter. It didn't have the same impact. They soon returned to the sexy standard.

But even if sex is as much an attention-getter for women as it is for men, do they process it in the same way? After all, genital response patterns vary between the sexes. Perhaps attention patterns vary too.

As it turns out, that's exactly the case – with data showing women don't just physically respond to categories of porn in a different way to men, they watch it differently too.

As far as sexual paraphernalia go, the eye-tracking device ranks low on consumer appeal. You'd never see it topping the sales figures at Ann Summers or featuring in a *Playboy* centrefold shoot. But as a tool for assessing attention and focus in test subjects, it's the Rampant Rabbit of the research world. Its importance is in being able to measure what people are looking at, and how long they look. With the combination of a laptop screen and an eye-tracking headset, experimenters can use software to determine where in a photo catches a test subject's attention and how long they spend looking at an image.

With a growing body of evidence to show that women and men do not respond to visual erotica in the same way – but that they do, definitely, respond – one intriguing question is, *what exactly are they looking at?* After all, the different results in what men and women find arousing might come from the different ways in which they are viewing and processing images.

A number of groups have looked into this area. Unfortunately, several of the studies did not use the same images when testing men and women, which makes the results impossible to compare. If you show women photos of naked vs clothed men, and show men pictures of naked vs clothed women, all that will demonstrate is whether people prefer to look at nudes (unsurprisingly, yes, that's exactly what they prefer).[7] It doesn't answer the question of how men and women respond to the *same* stimuli.

A research group in Atlanta set out to do just that. Digital photos of oral sex and intercourse were downloaded from the internet.

Researchers rated the photos for overall attractiveness to come up with seventy-two test images – the ones considered most attractive. Not a bad day's work in the lab, if you ask me.

Both men and women were recruited to look at the same set of photos. Participants were hooked up to the eye tracker while they looked at the seventy-two test images. They could look for as long as they liked before pressing a key to continue to the next. They were allowed to stop if they felt uncomfortable.

One interesting feature of this study is that women on hormonal birth control (HBC) were analysed separately from other women. Hormonal birth control, such as the pill, works by mimicking the state of the body in pregnancy, causing the ovaries to stop releasing eggs. The hormonal fluctuations that would ordinarily be experienced by women are dampened, and they show lower, less variable patterns of sexual motivation than women going through the natural cycle. If the body thinks it has already conceived, then the factors influencing sexual attraction will be significantly altered. This is something that has already long been noted in studies looking at differences in mate choice between HBC and non-HBC women. So what did the results show?

The researchers did not find much difference between men and both HBC and non-HBC women in how they subjectively rated each photo on attractiveness, nor did they find differences between men's and women's viewing times. This is inconsistent with the common myth that men find visual stimuli more engaging, since if you believed that, you would expect men to spend more time looking at the pictures. But what did differ were the areas of the images on which the men and women were focusing.

When comparing men, women on birth control, and women not on birth control, researchers noticed diverging patterns between the groups. Tracking eye movement over the screen revealed that men spent more time looking at female faces, and were more likely than either group of women to do so.[8]

But it was the non-HBC women, not the men, who had a truly roving eye. Those women who were not on birth control and therefore experiencing more natural hormonal influence had more first looks towards genitals. They also spent markedly more time looking at genitals, and not only that, were more likely than men to do so overall.

The HBC women's watching patterns showed that they spent more time looking at the clothes of the people in the images and at the background.

What do the differences between the men and non-HBC women tell us? Again, it goes back to the idea that while the external male body conveys sexual interest unambiguously, the clues as to whether a woman is turned on are more subtle. It could be that for heterosexual men, looking at the face of a woman is a better way of interpreting the level of sexual excitement than looking at her body. Is she naked and emotionally uninvolved, or is she 'up for it'? The face probably tells more about how interested a woman is than the naked body alone would. Women, on the other hand, don't need to see a man's face to know whether he's sexually ready, so they don't spend as much time looking there.

Not only does pornography of all varieties turn women on, but it also seems to address problems even pharmaceutical science can't touch.

An interesting bookend to the revelations about women and erotica is the parallel discussion about women's sex lives as they go through the menopause. It's an issue that relies heavily on stereotypes about women and lack of sexual desire. It also seems to exploit modern insecurities about having the 'right' kind of sex, having it often enough, and being perfectly satisfied at all times.

The 'problem' of female sexual dysfunction (FSD) has been a research holy grail for drug companies in recent years. It seems partly inspired by the runaway success of Viagra and Cialis, and partly by a new openness among women when it comes to talking about and pursuing good sex. And with people not only living longer lives but healthier ones too, the expectation of continuing to have fulfilling sex continues even after menopause in women.

However, no drug has emerged to transform female sexual response in the same way that Viagra has for men with erectile dysfunction. And it isn't as if the big pharmaceutical companies haven't tried. They have tested everything from giving Viagra to women to testosterone patch treatments and developing new drugs altogether, but success has been far from universal. The straightforward approach of increasing blood flow to the genitals or pumping the system with increased hormones doesn't seem to be the magic bullet for women in the way it is for men.

The pharmaceutical industry wields a lot of power. Companies that produce drugs maintain internal research units, fund outside academic activity, and supply sponsorship for conferences. When the pharmaceutical industry as a whole becomes interested in a particular topic, it has – far more than any scientists or patients on their own – the means to help direct where research attention goes.

Groups with this kind of impact can be thought of as Agenda Setters. Their interest can define the discussion, and their views on particular topics nudge others into action.

Agenda Setters needn't be companies or industries. They may be governments, NGOs (non-governmental organisations), religious groups, or charities. They are usually large, well funded, and well organised. Agenda Setters are anyone with a particular viewpoint and the resources to disseminate that viewpoint through experts to the general public. Often, they have a particular outcome in mind. That could range from selling certain products to pushing particular laws or furthering a specific ideology.

Now, what exactly is meant by an agenda? Usually, the agenda is a focus on money, political power, or morality. Often, all three: getting money, maintaining power, and enforcing morality. Why do the agendas exist? Mainly because they are financially and socially profitable. After all, the people involved in these activities are hardly volunteers. They are well remunerated, respected in certain circles, and influential.

At the risk of sounding a bit 'enemy of the state', I'd like to emphasise how the economic and social agenda differs from, say, the patriarchy conspiracy theory advanced by some feminists. Feminism has, like people who claim to have seen UFOs, correctly identified a phenomenon, but completely misappropriated its origin. The agendas at work here have nothing to do with Masonic secret societies or their like.

Rather, the agenda is the agenda of the schoolyard – getting to the top of the social heap and staying there. The rules are not coded in indecipherable hieroglyph and filed away in the depths of the Bodleian; they are obvious, popular, and widely accepted. And the tactics are simply the tactics of the schoolyard writ large.

The Agenda Setters interested in female libido have some impressive-sounding numbers to quote. In 1999, a paper in the *Journal of the American Medical Association* claimed to have uncovered a widespread phenomenon: that 43 per cent of women suffered from sexual dysfunction – in other words about 50 million American women. The author, sociologist Edward Laumann, based the conclusions on the results of a survey of 1800 women under the age of sixty.[9]

Laumann, of course, is not an Agenda Setter, but his paper could be used by them. The results he reported provided the impetus for a whole raft of research activity: activity that was, by and large, commissioned by and conducted for Pfizer, the manufacturers of Viagra, and other companies such as Procter & Gamble and Boehringer.

According to Ray Moynihan, a journalist who has written extensively about female sexual dysfunction in the *British Medical Journal* and in a recent book, 'The corporate-sponsored creation of a disease is not a new phenomenon, but the making of female sexual dysfunction is the freshest, clearest example we have.'[10] The Agenda Setters put their focus on women's sexual lives, and their agenda – to sell a cure – is clear.

One way to convince people they're unwell is to suggest a problem is widespread. A former manager for a company that worked on a hormonal vaginal cream, described it in the film *Orgasm Inc.* as 'kind of complicated, because you have to have a disease before you can treat it'. She even went so far as to admit, 'We've been able to get thought leaders involved in female sexual dysfunction, and really work closely with them to develop this disease entity, so that it makes sense.'[11]

'Developing' diseases in this way may even include manipulating the data as it is gathered. Asking questions about people experiencing acute symptoms in the recent past will get you far smaller numbers than asking about a range of symptoms occurring over time. Are pharmaceutical companies massaging the numbers to convince people they have something that might not exist?

The numbers from the original survey on the prevalence of FSD look high, but even in peer-reviewed research it's important not to simply take statements at face value. The results are from questions asking if the women had experienced pain or lack of desire at *any time in the previous year*. The rather high 43 per cent is actually a grand total ... not the proportion of women experiencing this on a regular basis. People who said they sometimes and seldom had problems were also included. 'When you look at the proportions of women experiencing these sexual difficulties "frequently", the numbers collapse,' says Ray Moynihan in his book.[12]

It's a bizarre sleight of hand to imply that if a woman, at any time and for any reason, lacks desire even once in a year, she has some kind of sexual desire disorder. And equating pain during intercourse – which could be due to all kinds of medical causes, or recent childbirth – with sexual dysfunction? It boggles the mind, it truly does.

Other studies have uncovered a gap between the number of women who can be potentially diagnosed with FSD and those who seem to actually have a problem. A study in London compared the newly developed diagnosis against the number of women who felt they experienced negative sexual dysfunction effects. While using the diagnostics found 38 per cent of women had sexual dysfunction, only 18 per cent of the women thought their symptoms concerning – and just 6 per cent rated it 'moderate' or 'severe'.[13] Surely, if there is a problem with lack of desire for sex, the best placed person to decide whether it's severe or not is the woman herself ... not some arbitrary clinical scale.

A Swedish study confirmed that less than half of women who reported decreased interest in sex over time considered themselves dissatisfied.[14] Another study by Irwin Nazareth in London looked at subjects recruited from GP surgeries and suggested that in people who could be diagnosed with a sexual dysfunction, 'reduced sexual interest or response may be a normal adaptation to stress.'[15] In other words, could what is being labelled as a disorder actually be a natural ebbing and flowing of desire over time?

What would be the reasons for such disagreement between the diagnoses and the number of people reporting problems? One reason could be that people were not discussing their problems with GPs – possible, but the Nazareth et al. study suggested that patients are pretty honest with their doctors when it comes to sexual difficulty. While it is plausible that people who speak to their GP about problems with sex are a self-selecting group, making the study an undercount of people with the syndrome, there is no easy way to correct this. As this book will explore later on, the 'dark art' of estimating unknown populations is a much misunderstood, and sometimes abused, approach to diagnosis.

Another reason could be that the criteria are defined too broadly. In some cases it looks like even an occasional event merits a scary diagnosis. But what would be the benefit of overdiagnosing the population? Some diagnostic manuals, such as the fourth edition of the *Diagnostic and Statistical Manual of Mental Disorders* (DSM-IV), have been criticised for possible conflict of interest between the committees who write the disease definitions and the pharmaceutical companies selling prescription drugs. Half of the people on the DSM committees have some kind of connection to a drug company. On the committees writing definitions for some areas of disorders, the figure shoots up to almost 100 per cent.[16]

Because of their controversial nature, there has been a push to reconsider the criteria for sexual dysfunction – considerations that may be reflected in the upcoming DSM-V. According to a paper by Richard Balon and Anita Clayton, 'Marked distress or interpersonal difficulty is a criterion of all DSM-defined sexual dysfunctions,'[17] since this helps determine what is and is not normal. But if large numbers of women being diagnosed say they are not distressed, then how can the diagnosis be real?

So it's unsurprising that drugs hyped as potential 'female Viagra' have not done well. Along with the failure of Viagra-like vasodilation drugs and hormone treatments, drugs that target neurotransmitters have also failed to have an effect. Procter & Gamble's experimental testosterone patch was rejected by the US Food and Drug Administration in December 2004. The German drug company Boehringer stopped developing its drug flibanserin after unsuccessful clinical trials in North America.[18]

The assumptions made by Agenda Setters and the researchers they influenced all follow old stereotypes. The drugs either try to increase vaginal blood flow (implied: women don't get turned on easily, so drug intervention is needed), or they try to boost testosterone (implied: women don't have hormones like men's, so drug intervention is needed). Others focus on neurotransmitters (implied: there's something lacking in women's brain chemistry, so drug intervention is needed).

Characterising natural variations in women's libidos as a problem that needs to be solved is nothing new. What is novel is the interest from big pharmaceutical companies and other Agenda Setters in getting involved on a commercial scale. In the 1966 book *Feminine Forever*, author Robert Wilson suggested that the menopause is a 'disease' of female hormone deficiency and that good sexual health could be saved by taking hormones. Wilson's writing was hugely influential. In the following decades, hormone replacement became a popular option for Western women above a certain age. It's a treatment that is far from cheap and demands constant upkeep, and has been linked with some negative side effects including cancer and heart disease.

Hormone replacement and its supposed benefits, particularly for older women's sex lives, however, are at odds with the experimental evidence. With their famously extensive laboratory research, Masters and Johnson showed in 1970 that 'nothing could be further from the truth than the oft-expressed concept that aging women do not maintain a high level of sexual orientation.' The menopause does cause thinning of the vaginal walls and decrease in lubrication, but the studies found no decrease in clitoral function, which is the real cause of orgasm.[19]

Undoubtedly there are women who do suffer from sexual problems, and over the course of a lifetime, this can affect a large proportion of people at some point or another. But claiming it's a disease in approximately half of all women all the time? Not only does this exploit old stereotypes about women and lack of desire, it's a strategy that hardly helps the smaller proportion of women who are distressed and might actually benefit from targeted and sensitive treatment.

The characterisation of variations in female libido as a dysfunction has not led to a pharmaceutical success. This hasn't stopped the interest of Agenda Setters, however – far from it.

The World Congress for Sexual Health, held in Glasgow in June 2011, attracted sexual health experts from all over the world. Papers presented at the conference were published in the prestigious *Journal of Sexual Medicine*. Alongside the research areas you might expect at the conference, like HIV prevention, teenage pregnancy, and gender and sexuality there was a session entirely devoted to 'Hypoactive sexual disorders among women and pharmacological treatments'. One of the major exhibitors supporting the conference was the drug company Bayer, which has been developing and marketing an intra-vaginal drug meant to treat (wait for it) ... female sexual dysfunction.

It's interesting to note that while the Agenda Setters press on with their pharmaceutical solution, research indicates there may be a real, and cheap, way to address the problem for those who are actually suffering.

Studies of treatments for FSD that only take a pharmaceutical approach have been negative or mixed. Studies that include erotic images, however, have been far more successful in getting results. Postmenopausal women on oestrogen-replacement treatments were treated with sildenafil (the generic name for Viagra) in an attempt to restore orgasmic ability.[20] While the drug on its own did not do much, the study also combined pharmaceutical treatment with watching porn. The paper notes that '[t]he erotic video significantly increased subjective sexual arousal in all women' but that they 'do not benefit from sildenafil'.

Or in other words, put a sexual context back into women's lives, stop harping on about a supposed dysfunction, and before you know it they may start to sexually respond. It's not really all that surprising, is it?

A pity for the Agenda Setters that they aren't in the business of producing porn films. Or at least, they aren't ... yet.

The power of sex and sexuality over our lives goes far beyond producing offspring. The reasons for this are far older than our society, older than humanity, even. Evolutionary theory suggests several main drivers of survival. Natural selection is one of the most well known. Natural selection says the traits that prevent death before maturity become more common in a species over time. This is because the individuals with the traits live long enough to pass it on to the next generation. For example, a variation that enables a moth to be camouflaged better, so predators can't see it, makes it more likely to live to reproduce and pass that gene on. The offspring that inherit the mutation will also benefit, and be more likely to continue reproducing.

But sexual selection is also important: from the cold point of view of animal reproduction, if you can't attract a mate, it hardly matters whether you made it to adulthood or not. The large horns of the male red deer, for example, are used not for gathering food or anything else related to day-to-day survival. They are used for the express purpose of fighting other males to impress, and thus gain access to, females. The elaborate feathers and mating dances of the male birds of paradise are an adaptation that serves a similar purpose. It doesn't affect whether they make it to adulthood, but it does make mating and procreation more likely for the genetically fortunate.

Natural selection and sexual selection can work together in the same species: the muted, camouflaging colouration of a pea hen is a result of natural selection because it keeps her safe. The male peacock's extravagant tail feathers are a result of sexual selection because it makes him attractive as a mate.

Until recently, the question of why humans evolved large brains and language abilities focused on natural selection. Our brains, as a percentage of our body volume, are much larger than those of our closest ape relatives. Scientists suggested that human brains grew in response to a need for greater cognitive skills, and that these were necessary for getting food. Language skills were attributed to a need for aiding co-operation (and therefore survival) within a family group.

However, some have started to ask whether the size of our brains is actually the result not of natural selection, but sexual selection. After all, relying on natural selection alone does not address very much of what makes us human. The abilities of creating music and appreciating literature, for example, don't give much advantage in hunting food, avoiding predators, or seeking shelter. You don't need art to reach puberty.

But when such adaptations are recast as developments in the eternal race to attract and mate, some of the human abilities that are unnecessary in the day-to-day survival world of the caveman begin to make sense.

Geoffrey Miller poses an interesting question in his book *The Mating Mind: How Sexual Choice Shaped the Evolution of Human Nature.*[21]

'Why omit sexual desire and sexual choice from the pantheon of evolutionary forces that could have shaped the human mind, when biologists routinely use sexual choice to explain behavioural abilities in other animals?'

Not only does he make a thought-provoking point, it is a point that considers women to be equally as involved in sexual choice as men are. Women have aptitude for music, art, language, and every other non-survival adaptation humans have developed, just as men do. If they weren't as interested as men were in mating but adapted merely to survive, surely they would be less like the flamboyant peacock and more like the poor pea hen: drab, dull, hiding in the undergrowth while she waits to be won.

Of course, as with most theories in the young field of evolutionary biology, it's an idea that is very speculative and hotly contested. It's only an idea. In order to prove it, far more research would need to be done from many different areas of the scientific spectrum, and even then it may never be confirmed whether the truth is one or the other (or both, or neither). But it is food for thought when considering women's interest in sex. Particularly when many have long assumed women's interest in sex is strictly tied to security and child rearing.

Sex is a powerful social glue. People who suppress or are incapable of having children still have rich and active sex lives. Postmenopausal women still want to, and do, experience sexual feelings. The abundance of reliable birth control methods does not eliminate the desire to have sex.

We are not the only species where the female sex drive is about more than just procreation. The bonobo, which along with the chimpanzee is our closest relative in the animal kingdom, has what can only be described as a wild sex life.

Bonobos were formerly known as pygmy chimpanzees. For a long time they were assumed to be the same species as chimps, and were only recognised as a separate species in 1933. One of the more well-documented differences between chimps and bonobos is their behaviour ... specifically, their sexual behaviour.

One of the many things bonobos and humans share is the pursuit of sex even when procreation is not possible. Couplings between the same sex are widely observed in bonobo communities, as well as sex with individuals too old to reproduce. Interestingly, this happens in both bonobos and humans even when procreative, heterosexual sex is possible and available.

Another similarity with humans is that sex is also integrated into the natural social life of the species. In *Sexual Nature, Sexual Culture*, author Paul Abramson records in great detail the varieties and frequencies of sexual acts among bonobos.[22]

Other apes like gorillas and chimpanzees mate in the ventro-dorsal, or 'doggy style', position. But bonobos, like humans, also like to copulate face-to-face. Mouth kissing and mutual masturbation are frequent activities with bonobos, just as they are with us. Fellatio and cunnilingus happen frequently, as do male-male and female-female genital rubbing. And the activity is not necessarily just a reproduction strategy. While sexual activity is far more frequent in bonobos than in chimpanzees, the fertility rate for the two species is about the same.

The status of the females in bonobo society is more equal than it is in chimpanzee society, and females can control food access. Trading sex for food occurs regularly between bonobo females, appears to reduce tension, and aids co-operation. These encounters lead to stable long-term relationships between females. This in turn helps them form coalitions, control resources, and elevate their status.[23] This is as true for bonobos in the wild as it is for their counterparts in captivity.[24]

Sexual activity seems to fulfil an important social function in bonobo groups, particularly among females, who initiate more sex than the males and have more same-sex interaction. Sex is more frequent around feeding time and after a fight, suggesting it helps maintain friendly relationships. Bonobos do not form permanent sexual partnerships and, with the exception of mothers and sons abstaining from sex together, do not discriminate in types of partners. When bonobos discover a new food source, this usually leads to communal sex, which appears to decrease tension and encourage peaceful feeding in the group.

While it is still debated whether bonobos are matriarchal or not, it is agreed that female bonobos are not subordinate to males, unlike female chimpanzees. And unlike chimpanzees (and, for that matter, humans) there have been no observations of lethal aggression among bonobos either in the wild or in captivity.

Sexual acts clearly serve an important purpose in bonobo society and females instigate this activity more frequently than males do. That all of this occurs in one of the species most closely related to humans should hardly come as a surprise.

Maybe Freud would have had a better chance of understanding female desire if he had sat a few apes on that couch instead of people.

This picture of the social, sexual bonobo female with wide-ranging tastes and desires is starting to be reflected in human studies as well. Not only with the studies examining pornography viewing and genital arousal in women, but also in terms of how relationships are formed.

Scientists who study sexual orientation have found that there is a difference in the patterns of male and female sexual orientation. Women's sexuality appears to be more fluid, and less categorical. This is interesting considering that the studies of male and female differences in physiological arousal showed similar results.

Women are more likely to have shifted in sexual orientation during their lives than men are. For women, same- or opposite-sex relationships are less likely to have been an exclusive state.[25] Studies suggest a lot of difference between the origins of homosexual feeling in gay men and gay women, with more gay men reporting their first attractions to be a result of physical arousal, but women being more likely to have had their first same-sex experiences as the result of a 'passionate friendship'.[26]

Dr Lisa Diamond from the University of Utah, who tracks how women categorise their sexuality over time, observed that in every two years up to 30 per cent of participants in her studies change how they label their sexual identity. Over longer observation, about 70 per cent change how they described themselves at their initial interview.[27]

There are plenty of high-profile examples of women who were previously married to men coming out as lesbians in later life. Women such as Cynthia Nixon, who plays Miranda in *Sex and the City*, or Mary Portas from *Mary Queen of Shops* have given high visibility to the phenomenon of the 'late-life lesbian'.

Dr Diamond speculated why this might happen. 'In my study, what I often found was that women who may have always thought that other women were beautiful and attractive would, at some point later in life, actually fall in love with a woman.' It wasn't that they'd been repressing their true desires before, though. Rather, without the context of an actual relationship, the occasional fantasies women had earlier in their sexual lives just weren't considered that significant to their partner choice.'[28]

Rather than assume older women who come out as gay or bi were suppressing their true desires for decades, Diamond's research suggests that multiple possibilities exist all along. Women seem to respond as much to the particular qualities of the partner in question as they do to specific gender.

While more research focuses on gay men instead of gay women, the origin of sexual orientation in women appears to have a different basis to that of men.[29] There are numerous studies comparing gay men to straight men. They show measurable differences in things like handedness, brain structure, and sensitivity to particular pheromones. Whether this is due to genetics, developmental environment, or some combination of the two is unclear. But, nevertheless, the biological differences in gay and straight men seem to be consistent across a wide range of research.

Where these studies have been performed on women, the differences between women who are straight and those who are bisexual or gay is less clear than it is for men. The rigid stereotype of the excessively masculine lesbian is sometimes true, but it's not the norm. Whether this is due to a different mix of genetic or environmental factors is uncertain. But it does show it's possible that male homosexuality and female homosexuality originate in completely different ways.

Just because women can and do change, of course, does not make that a basis for discrimination. Many opponents of homosexuality have used such research to claim that one 'chooses' whether to be homosexual, like picking a meal off a menu. Dr Diamond has been very critical of that simplistic viewpoint in interviews: 'I think the culture tends to lump together change and choice, as if they're the same phenomenon, but they're not. Puberty involves a heck of a lot of change, but you don't choose it.'[30] And with humans having same-sex coupling and sexual fluidity in common with our closest ape relatives, it seems reasonable to think of it as at least partly the result of evolution, rather than something a few people have fashionably (if you believe the cynics) 'chosen'.

As the studies of physical response to erotica demonstrate, it turns out women respond physically to a far broader range of sexual stimuli than men do. Even women who identify themselves as straight can be polymorphously perverse, to borrow the Freudian phrase – capable of erotic attachment with, well, anyone.

In fact a lot of the results give renewed credibility to Freud's notion of innate bisexuality, the idea that humans are born bisexual but through psychological development eventually settle with an orientation, with the bisexuality remaining in a latent state. Later, the research of Alfred Kinsey took the idea a step further, proposing a continuum of human sexuality that stretches between heterosexuality and homosexuality rather than discrete, unchanging categories.

Other ways of considering sexuality exist as well. Gore Vidal once suggested, 'There is no such thing as homosexuality or heterosexuality; there are only homosexual and heterosexual acts.' The sexual life of bonobos would appear to support this as another possibility.

And, of course, there are many examples of people whose sexuality evades established definitions. This doesn't mean their sexuality doesn't exist but rather that we don't yet have appropriate words to describe their sexual lives. We may never have.

It's clear the capacity for high sexual appetite in females and a wide variety of sexual pairings is something we share with our closest animal relatives. When combined with recent research results, and increased visibility of late-life lesbian couples, this suggests that visible female sexuality and having both male and female partners is not an aberration for women. In fact, it is perfectly natural.

But it's important to remember that sexual arousal and sexual interest are not the same thing. If they were, one might conclude from the studies that women would rather have sex with animals than humans, or that most heterosexual women are only somewhat attracted to heterosexual men! Clearly, that's not the case. We can't assume emotional attachment is irrelevant to attraction, but for too long it has been assumed that in the case of women, emotional attachment is all there is. The research shows that is not true.

What is especially interesting about this area is what it adds to the picture of female sexuality. There are loads of theories about what women want: everything from old men with fast cars to young studs with a nifty line in housework. And some of the most profitable companies on the planet have turned their gaze towards female sexuality, with less than impressive results. But the real story is far more primal, and interesting, than any of those approaches would predict.

As with so many myths, there is a flipside. For every stereotype of the sexually undermotivated female, there is a supposedly sexually rampant male. For every prim and modest woman, there is someone whose sexuality is dark, threatening, and dangerous. For every Eve, a Lilith. Unsurprisingly, this oversimplification of human sexuality has led to the rise of another voguish idea – that of sex addiction.

2

MYTH: Sex addiction is a real psychological disorder, and it's on the increase.

W hat did you have for breakfast this morning? Was it a fry-up? Toast and jam? Yoghurt and fruit, or simply a black coffee before rushing out the door?

Or did you have a bowl of flakes instead? Corn flakes, perhaps, or bran? Because, if so, your breakfast is at the very cutting edge of what is scientifically known about preventing sexual addiction …

… in the nineteenth century, that is.

John Harvey Kellogg didn't invent the first dry breakfast cereal, but he was one of the earliest and most successful manufacturers of it. What most people don't realise is that the Kellogg's cereals that we still have on supermarket shelves today were the result of one man's moral and sexual beliefs.

Kellogg was a member of the Seventh-Day Adventist Church and advocated sexual abstinence. He wrote books explaining his approach, called *Plain Facts about Sexual Life* and *Plain Facts for Old and Young.* His belief was that a bland and balanced diet consisting of two meals a day would promote all sorts of health benefits, chief among these being a reduction in sexual feelings. He believed that anyone experiencing sexual temptation should avoid stimulating food and drinks, and eat no meat. To Kellogg, the suppression of sexual desire was a matter of life and death, particularly when it came to the 'solitary vice' of masturbation – a vice he believed would eventually result in death, where 'Such a victim literally dies by his own hand.'

The notion that eating a bowl of Frosties could save people from physical and psychological damage was hardly unique to Kellogg. In the nineteenth century it was widely believed that people in general, and particularly women, were susceptible to harm from being over-stimulated and giving in to their urges.

Belief in the danger of excessive sexual desire became especially voguish after publication of *Nymphomania, or a Dissertation Concerning the Furor Uterinus*, written by MDT Bienville and translated into English in 1775. French physician Bienville discussed how rich food, chocolate, impure thoughts, reading novels, and masturbation overstimulated nerve fibres and led to nymphomania.

But if restricting yourself to plain crackers and dry flakes sounds terrible, it was nothing compared to some of the more aggressive medical treatments available.

One particularly detailed case study dates from 1841. Miss T, a twenty-nine-year-old farmer's daughter, was diagnosed with nympho-mania. According to a report by her doctors in the *Boston Medical and Surgical Journal*, she exhibited all the telltale signs of a nymphoma-niac: she was restless, her vagina moist, and she had a tumid clitoris. A nurse reported her body wracked with a 'paroxysm of hysteria' – or what we today would more commonly call an orgasm.[31] She was given stool softeners, opium, and muriatic acid as a first course of treatment.

When she did not respond, Miss T was given a solution of lead to induce vomiting. A blistering agent was applied to the base of her neck. Treatment for this serious illness was harsh, but it was widely thought such measures were more than justified in these cases. Caustic potash was applied to her genitals. This was supposed to lessen their sensitiv-ity (and, after the considerable burns, probably did exactly that).

Treatment for women like Miss T would also have included bleed-ing. This might have involved putting leeches on the perineum – the skin between the vaginal and anal openings – to draw off blood. The report notes that 'twenty ounces of blood [were] abstracted', though it does not say how. The barbarity of the treatment led to apparently suc-cessful results. After several weeks, the patient was greatly improved, with 'not a symptom remaining referable to nymphomania'. She now demonstrated 'every appearance of modesty' and her 'sphincter and vagina generally much contracted'.

The idea of the sex-crazed woman wasn't new to the eighteenth and nineteenth centuries. Ancient Greece had the *maenads*, crazed and drunken female followers of Dionysus. Ancient Rome had stories about women like Claudius's wife, Messalina, the 'whore-empress' (according to Juvenal) who supposedly bested a famous prostitute in a sex competition. But these were unusual examples, the highly sexed actions considered rare aberrations from a woman's 'natural' urges. And quite apart from that, the tales were also probably untrue.

Victorian doctors (and society in general) believed that sexual desire in a woman was a symptom of disease. Gynaecological problems were thought to be the main source of both physical and mental disorders in women. These were treated with approaches like the ones described for the case of Miss T. Others received surgery like clitoridectomy (removal of the clitoris) or ovariotomy (removal of the ovaries).

When women approached doctors with concern about their desires, physicians saw the potential for severe nymphomania. Even behaviour as mild as a lascivious glance could be suspect. Women who did not respond to treatment might be put in a mental institution. From that point on, their conditions often worsened.

The reports of nymphomaniacs in asylums were shocking – physical attacks, obscene language, violent masturbation. Increasingly this was seen not as an unusual result of extreme treatment and incarceration, but as a possible outcome for *any* unchecked female libido.

The treatment of Miss T, even the use of leeches and acid, was not unusual for that time. The causes of disease were unknown, so doctors relied on remedies last updated in ancient Greece. They thought disease came from the body being out of balance. Bloodletting and burning were supposed to bring back equilibrium. Cold water, sedatives, and – yes – a mild diet consisting of breakfast cereals were supposed to produce positive, calming results.

'After much soul searching, I have decided to take an indefinite break from professional golf,' Tiger Woods announced in a press release on his website in December 2009. 'I need to focus my attention on being a better husband, father, and person.'

The announcement followed revelations of the golf player's private life, in particular his numerous affairs. In spite of being married with children, Woods also pursued sex with glamorous women, models, and hostesses. Woods cited sexual addiction as the cause of his straying and promptly checked in to a treatment centre in Mississippi.

Tiger Woods isn't the only celebrity name to have been linked with sex addiction. *X-Files* actor David Duchovny has sought treatment for sex addiction; 80s rocker Rick Springfield admitted to a time in his life feeling that sex was 'the thing that you use to make you feel good'; Billy Bob Thornton; Russell Brand; Michael Douglas – Hollywood gossip is not always to be believed but all have reportedly sought treatment for their private peccadilloes. But apparently, if the numbers are also to be believed, celebrities are not the only ones at risk. According to the National Association of Sexual Addiction Problems, 6–8 per cent of adults are sex addicts.

'I am deeply aware of the disappointment and hurt that my infidelity has caused to so many people, most of all my wife and children,' Woods said in his public statement before entering treatment. 'I want to say again to everyone that I am profoundly sorry and that I ask forgiveness. It may not be possible to repair the damage I've done, but I want to do my best to try.'

'Sex addiction', however, is not a term used as an official diagnosis in the American Psychiatric Association's *Diagnostic and Statistical Manual* (DSM-IV), considered the definitive word on psychological disorders.

'Hypersexuality' is the term the DSM-IV now uses that is closest in definition to what has historically been known as nymphomania in women and satyriasis in men. The World Health Organization's International Classification of Diseases (ICD-10), however, still lists nymphomania and satyriasis as subdivisions of the diagnosis 'excessive sexual drive'.[32]

In both cases, the terms refer to a desire to engage in sex at a level that is considered 'abnormally high' and 'causes distress'. It is characterised by a hyperactive sex drive and lowered sexual inhibitions. In the ICD-10 it falls under the category of 'Sexual dysfunction, not caused by organic disorder or disease', but the specific diagnostic protocol are unclear. Is this then the 'sexual addiction' talked about so much in the press and, if so, are celebrities like Tiger Woods especially susceptible?

There are groups such as Sexaholics Anonymous, Sex and Love Addicts Anonymous, and Sexual Addicts Anonymous. These groups are very popular and they do appear to help many people find some relief from their problems. But outside of the self-organising twelve-step groups, sexual addiction is also a multi-million-dollar industry. There are books and websites, treatment centres and programmes, and of course private therapists advising concerned clients. Many people benefit from this concept, even though there is debate about whether or not it exists.

In his book *Tabloid Medicine: How the Internet Is Being Used to Hijack Medical Science for Fear and Profit*, Robert Goldberg, PhD, explains how these and similar suspect 'syndromes' are created. Turns out, the 'manufactroversies', or controversies motivated by profit or ideology to intentionally create public confusion about an issue, all follow strikingly similar patterns described in Goldberg's book.

First, a new problem is created by redefining terminology. For example, what used to be commonly thought of as serial cheating or poor impulse control or just a bad husband is redefined as a 'sex addiction'. The redefinition creates the appearance of a surge in cases, since they will have gone from zero to everywhere, seemingly over-night. The beneficiaries? Pharmaceutical companies, or anyone else with a health-related public agenda. In other words ... Agenda Setters.

Then, self-appointed experts claim they have unique insight into the cause of the problem. And, in some cases, the experts have a financial interest in promoting their point of view, such as books, grants, or treatments.

The next step is when the media gets interested. They need new stories, and want to be the first to break news. The pressure for reporting an exclusive, coupled with underfunded reporting, means they often relay information – sometimes directly from PR releases – without checking the facts. And once something has been in the news, people assume it's credible, and that the media have done the fact checking for them. People who have heard the message often enough start to reframe their own behaviour according to these new definitions. Where before someone might have been just a cheating jerk, he now can claim to be suffering from 'narcissistic personality disorder' or a 'sex addiction'.

There is no denying that at least some of the people claiming a sex addiction are experiencing dangerous or worrying behaviour. Labels are useful, and have their place. Defining terms for alcoholism and drug addiction, for instance, helps give a framework where genuinely self-destructive and antisocial behaviour can be addressed. Step One of any twelve-step programme involves simply acknowledging that a problem exists. But is a fidelity problem *always* the same thing as an addiction? A rich guy cheating on his wife, that's a tragedy for the family, for sure. But are we calling someone an addict who is really just the equivalent of a social drinker, or an unpleasant drunk? There's a line that gets crossed in addictions, and it's a pretty extreme one. I've lived with addicts and I've lived with cheaters. There is no comparison.

In Chinese there is a saying:: 三人成虎 (sān rén chéng hǔ). Roughly translated, it means 'three men make a tiger'. The idea is that once you've heard about something from three different people, you're likely to take the story as truth without any other evidence. It only takes a handful of persuasive voices to convince people that something exists, even if it may not.

One of the people most influential in the area of 'sexual addiction' is Dr Patrick Carnes, who co-founded the Gentle Path sex addiction programme at the Mississippi treatment centre that Woods entered. Since 1992 he has written seven books on the topic and numerous articles. He wrote the definition of sexual addiction for the *Comprehensive Textbook of Psychiatry*, and established the treatment protocol.

His Wikipedia page also notes that he was awarded the distinguished Lifetime Achievement Award of the Society for the Advancement of Sexual Health, a society he co-founded in 1987.

On his website, Carnes gives a more explanatory definition of sexual addiction than either the DSM-IV or the ICD-10. He begins by saying that it is not about a single behaviour. But he does confirm that it includes some, and/or all, of the following: 'compulsive masturbation, compulsive heterosexual and homosexual relationships, pornography, prostitution, exhibitionism, voyeurism, indecent phone calls, child molesting, incest, rape and violence.'

Undoubtedly child molesting, incest, rape, and violence are wrong and should be causes for concern, regardless of whether they happen once or repeatedly. But surely those should be addressed by criminal law. And putting masturbation in the same category? Isn't that a little ... nineteenth-century thinking?

So, while some of the behaviours Carnes lists are clearly worrying, they are also extremely varied, perhaps too varied to fall under the same diagnostic umbrella. Is masturbation really somehow related to child molestation? If so, Carnes doesn't say how. Nor am I aware of any scientific evidence to suggest that this is the case.

Carnes developed the Sexual Addiction Screening Test, a diagnostic tool that aims to assess behaviour that may indicate a sex addiction. (It's unusual, even in a newly defined psychological disorder, for one person to have contributed so much to the definition and the diagnosis, not to mention the treatment criteria.)

The diagnostic test is disconcerting at times. Consider, for instance, a few yes-or-no questions:

Do you hide some of your sexual behaviours from others?

Has sex (or romantic fantasies) been a way for you to escape your problems?

Because the answers are yes or no, there's no room for interpretation. For instance, the child of very conservative parents may well hide sexual behaviours. Hiding your homosexuality from homophobes, in the narrow way the question is phrased, could potentially indicate you are a sex addict. And asking whether anyone has used fantasy as a way to escape problems ... isn't that more or less the definition of a fantasy?

Other questions address things that are increasingly acceptable to many people, and probably done by most. 'Have you spent considerable time surfing pornography online?' Since porn accounts for a large amount of paid content available online, then yes, you can assume a lot more people do it than are willing to be called addicts. Also, how much is 'considerable' time? Ten minutes? An hour? Ten hours? Without a guideline as to what the terminology means, it's ripe for inflation and misinterpretation by its users.

Ditto 'Have you regularly engaged in sadomasochistic behaviour?' Hmm – does anyone care to define what is meant by 'regularly'? Are we talking once a year, or once a day? I mean, is a gift pair of handcuffs on Valentine's Day the slippery slope to residential treatment? Or is there even a definition for what the test considers 'sadomasochistic'? One person's saucy spank is another person's hard-core kink. As with the criticism of female sexual dysfunction studies, it pays to be sceptical of data collection that relies on broad generalisations and ill-defined categories of severity.

Other questions in the self-assessment quiz seem to come across, perhaps unwittingly, as judging activities that most people would consider normal and not necessarily sexual. 'Have you used the internet to make romantic or erotic connections with people online?' Now, there's a question that risks judging the millions of people who have found fulfilling relationships via the internet and labelling them as addicts. And why the internet is singled out for special attention is unclear. People have been finding ways to date and mate with strangers since well before the world wide web.

But asking these questions about online interaction specifically feeds into the impression many articles give of sex addiction as a 'new' or 'emerging' phenomenon. There's no reason that would be true. After all, sex isn't new; availability of multiple partners isn't new. Why would sex addiction be any newer than alcoholism? Suggesting that internet technology and other modern accoutrements might be a source of the syndrome does not make sex addiction more plausible. That would be like saying alcoholism only exists because of off-licences.

Other questions seem likely to cause distress: 'Have you stayed in romantic relationships after they became emotionally or physically abusive?' I was once in an emotionally abusive relationship for years. My reasons for staying had nothing to do with sex and everything to do with fear. People stay in abusive relationships for all kinds of reasons, and I doubt those reasons are erotic. How does the crippling fear of leaving an abuser make someone a sex addict?

My favourite, clearly, is the question that asks, 'Have you been paid for sex?'

That makes no sense. Since when does being paid for something equate to a pathological obsession with it? You wouldn't screen people with suspected eating disorders by asking, 'Have you ever been a waitress?' You wouldn't suss out potential alcoholics by asking if they had ever worked behind a bar.

Another problem is that the test doesn't specify if you're meant to give answers about what you do now, or about what has ever happened in the past. It doesn't distinguish between happened before and happening now. Hands up who has ever walked out of a sexual encounter unfulfilled, or regretted a particular choice of partner. Isn't that part of learning about life and relationships? Answer the questions in the broadest way possible and we're probably all sex addicts.

The test has its flaws, but with so much celebrity endorsement of the condition's existence, plenty of people don't question the validity of the diagnosis. Diagnosing sex addiction might be interpreted by some as pathologising what is probably, to most of us, reasonable sexual behaviour. There is nothing particularly telling or even unusual about having a varied sex life or a rocky relationship history.

I've no doubt the questionnaire was written with the best possible intentions. But the reasoning behind many of the questions is unclear. There's nothing in general sexuality research literature proving any connection between some of the behaviours described and addiction. The questions are so wide open, the diagnosis is probably a matter of interpretation rather than an objective judgement. It's not hard to imagine how people using a self-diagnosis tool like this could be convinced they have a syndrome that they might not have. It's also not hard to imagine unscrupulous others looking to misuse the tool to make money out of the emotionally vulnerable or the rich and famous.

Scientific evidence for the last half-century has shown that addiction is rooted in distinct brain changes, like other mental illnesses such as depression. Cycles of desire and reward affect the circuitry of behaviour, emotion, and memory. However, there is no scientific evidence showing sex addiction to be, like alcoholism is, a primary, chronic disease. That may be because it's very new. Or it may be because evidence proving its existence to that level would be all but impossible to obtain. And certainly the tools now available would not be sufficient to give the syndrome indisputable diagnostic weight.

As a postgraduate student, I kept a toy hanging above my desk. It was a little wooden saw. I kept it there as a helpful reminder of one of the more useful sayings once common in computer programming: *To someone who only has a hammer, every problem looks like a nail.* The saw was there as a reminder never to rely on just a hammer.

Unfortunately, the widespread popularity of such tools – and their increased acceptance – makes it difficult for researchers of mental phenomena to diversify their toolboxes.

According to Allen Frances, MD, an emeritus professor at Duke University, 'Periodically, the media becomes obsessed with one or another celebrity … the latest example is the Tiger Woods media frenzy which will likely lead to an "epidemic" of "sexual addiction".'[33]

This commentary is not from a lay person, or even a minor figure in psychiatry, but the chair of the DSM-IV task force. In other words, by the person best placed to understand how and why disorders are included in diagnostic manuals, and the potential problems of inclusion.

According to Professor Frances, 'false epidemics' inspired by celebrity misfortunes come and go. People don't change very much or very quickly, but trends in what is considered 'normal' can and do. And he has stated concerns that hypersexuality is tipped to be the hot 'false epidemic' of the not so distant future.

But if psychiatry is a branch of medical science, how could this be the case? Surely the diagnostic criteria must be evidence based? Professor Frances says not always. 'There are no objective tests in psychiatry – no X-ray, laboratory, or exam that says definitively that someone does or does not have a mental disorder.' This means that what is diagnosed as a mental disorder could be influenced by professional and social forces. And with the distinction between mental disorders and 'normality' so fluid, rates of disorder diagnosis can rise easily.

According to National Institute of Mental Health (NIMH) estimates, a quarter of the US population – that's 60 million people – has a diagnosable mental disorder at any one time. That doesn't mean they necessarily *have* one, just that they could be diagnosed with one, if the judging criteria were stringently applied. One study found that by the age of thirty, 50 per cent of the population met the criteria for an anxiety disorder. Another 40 per cent could be diagnosed as depressed, and a third as alcohol dependent. 'In this brave new world of psychiatric overdiagnosis,' says Professor Frances, 'will anyone get through life without a mental disorder?'

And in the brave new world of sexual openness and celebrity

obsessions, will anyone get through life without a sexual disorder?

Professor Frances is not the only person concerned about the creation of possibly bogus diagnoses. Lynn Payer, in her book *Disease-mongers*,[34] identifies a checklist of tactics commonly used to create suspect 'disorders'. How does sexual addiction stand up to her criteria?

The first dodgy tactic she discusses is 'taking a normal function and implying that there's something wrong with it and it should be treated'. And sure enough, right on the front page of one popular self-diagnosis website, we see statements like 'Even the healthiest forms of human sexual expression can turn into self-defeating behaviors.'

Another questionable strategy Payer highlights is 'imputing suffering that isn't necessarily there'. Implying that you could have the symptoms but not know about them is one way of doing this – again on the same website, we have 'Often sexual addicts don't know what is wrong with them.'

Next, Payer flags up 'defining as large a proportion of the population as possible as suffering from the "disease"'. In 1991, it was estimated 3–6 per cent of the US adult population would have sex addiction.[35] That would be at least 7 million Americans and a minimum of 1.35 million Britons. If this were a fatal disease, such a high percentage of the population being affected would qualify as a Centers for Disease Control 'Category 5 epidemic' – the highest category that exists.

The scientific origin of that estimate is unclear, but has been repeated so often – even in peer-reviewed papers – that it is taken as fact. Even papers you expect might apply some analysis to the frequency of the disorder, such as one titled 'The epidemiology and phenomenology of compulsive sexual behavior',[36] repeat the percentage exactly as it was originally stated. It is difficult to find a single paper that has any population-based justification for the estimate. That's not epidemiology. That's pulling numbers out of thin air.

How about how the 'disease' is defined? According to one of these popular self-diagnosis websites, 'There is a growing body of evidence that early child abuse, especially sexual, is a primary factor in the onset of sex addiction.' It goes on to guess that abuse leads to biological changes in the brain that heighten arousal mechanisms. That's ... well, that's just a bizarre claim.

No specific evidence is cited to support the claim. What is

interesting, though, is the striking similarity with nineteenth-century beliefs regarding nymphomania. 'Diseased ovaries or disordered menstruation, gynaecologists argued, could lead to injury of the nervous system and of the brain and thus to mental illness.'[37]

There are many experts who are sceptical of the existence of sexual addiction. There is also debate about whether – even in the cases of alcohol and drug abuse – the addiction model we are used to is really an appropriate way of thinking about how, and why, people do things.

So why is so much written about sex addiction in the general media, and why is the coverage so uncritical?

The reasons for this may be to do with the nature of journalism. Many of the people who write about science are not themselves scientists, and even fewer are educated in the relevant field. They are limited by deadlines and column inches. Something that is straightforward to explain (most people know little about biochemistry) is a more attractive proposition than something that is complex.

If you tell people brain chemicals are involved, even if they don't understand the mechanisms specifically, the idea is at least graspable. It is like the 'problem' of female sexual dysfunction being something that is supposedly 'cured' by the liberal application of hormones. But trying to tell people the causes are unknown and multifactorial, and that the existence of the disorder is not even really confirmed? Good luck getting that across in thirty seconds at the end of the local news.

According to experts, 'Even reductionist theories of mental illness such as of depression and schizophrenia seek to account for a general state of mind, not specific behaviour.'[38] So why are addictions believed to be down to a single factor, a kind of irresistible spell that if only we had the one single treatment key, we could master for good?

More to the point, isn't putting sex in this category – a single and powerful cause of ruin – simply a more modern version of the Devil putting temptations in our path to mislead and ruin us?

These kinds of concerns about sex addiction, and related ones about the prevalence of porn, are also proving big business in some Christian churches in the US. Books targeted at that community, such as *Healing the Wounds of Sexual Addiction* and *Eyes of Integrity: The Porn Pandemic and How It Affects You,* sell in the hundreds of thousands.

According to some of these books, sexual sin – which includes masturbation and any thoughts about sex outside of actually having sex with one's spouse – is a temptation that must be resisted at all costs. They emphasise that any of these actions result in lack of intimacy in marriage, and go against the biblical mandate to get and stay married.

But books aren't the only option on the menu. Consider Pure Life Ministries, a 44-acre 'porn recovery' retreat in western Kentucky where treatment is $175 per week for six to twelve months, and wives aren't allowed to visit. Since most participants quit their jobs to relocate to the centre, it's hard to imagine how this strengthens a marriage.

Or accountability2you, a service that dumps all the porn someone downloads into their spouse's email inbox, as an incentive to abstain. A similar product from XXXChurch.com offers porn-detection software that automatically emails a 'faith buddy' with your transgressions. All for only $7 a month.

While it's not uncommon for the people running such programmes to have sexual addiction counselling certification from the American Association of Christian Counselors, many are not licensed by the American Psychological Association.

Even within the Christian community, there are doubts about the diagnoses popping up thick and fast among congregations. Dr Mark Laaser, who has counselled Christians on sex matters since the 1980s, criticises such 'pray it away' groups. 'The field of addiction is much deeper than opening your Bible,' he said in a CNN interview. 'One affair doesn't mean you're a porn addict. Looking at porn occasionally doesn't make you a porn addict. Those may be poor decisions, but they are not necessarily caused by clinical addiction.'[39]

And yet there are many voices, not just those of the authors of books on addiction, supporting the sex addiction treatment process. They say they've been through it, and that the treatment works. What gives?

Doctors in the eighteenth and nineteenth centuries reported success with their treatment of their unnamed nymphomania patients. And now, certainly many people seem to feel some benefit from putting a name – sex addiction – to their behaviour and going through some kind of therapy for it.

But just because people claim that something works doesn't mean it works in the way they think. Treatment is comforting. I have trouble sleeping from time to time; I find baths help. Feeling better after a hot bath doesn't mean the bath 'cured' anything in and of itself. I was not suffering from a deficiency of hot water. It seems more likely the bath is a kind of displacement activity that makes me feel less anxious, so I can go to sleep.

Whether it's medical intervention or therapy, people seem to improve when they think something is being done. This is powerful and not to be dismissed; we know it as the placebo effect. A pill that contains no active ingredients can produce a result in some patients, if they simply believe that it will work. Power of positive thinking and all that.

Without doubt, for nineteenth-century middle-class women diagnosed as mild nymphomaniacs, talking to someone about their thoughts and having a cool bath was very reassuring. But that approach – and the more extreme treatments that could follow – seems to have done little for the cases observed in institutions, where there was probably a severe and underlying disorder at work.

The National Association of Sexual Addiction Problems says, 'Most [sex] addicts do not break the law, nor do they satisfy their need by forcing themselves upon others.' Respected sex therapist Marty Klein says, 'It's important to remind people that feeling out of control is not the same as being out of control.' Surely if many of the so-called sex addicts were truly uncontrollable, we'd be reading 'Tiger Woods convicted of assault' instead of 'Tiger Woods, cheater'.

If sex addiction appears not to have a diagnostic basis, then why do things like the DSM-IV designation for hypersexuality exist at all?

Perhaps because unmanageable sexual urges do exist, although far more rarely than in 6 per cent of the population, and rarely in isolation from other disorders. For example, there are people with mental disorders, and sometimes, other physiological conditions, who express sexual desire far beyond the boundaries of what is considered normal. This is quite different in degree to your average cheater. Even a very prolific one.

A friend of mine once worked as a nurse in a care home for young people with Prader-Willi syndrome. Prader-Willi is a genetic disorder, caused by a partial deletion of chromosome 15. Features of the syndrome include a host of physical characteristics, as well as learning difficulties, speech and sleeping disorders, and most markedly, polyphagia – overeating to an extreme degree. And extreme doesn't mean 'Oops, I finished all the ice cream, tee hee.' She described how the home could not even have scented soap, as the patients might think it smelled like food, and eat it. Food cupboards were naturally locked and monitored. The residents literally could not help themselves.

She also told me about some encounters with residents who had trouble understanding what was and was not sexually appropriate. There were patients she had to remind not to masturbate in public, not to say whatever sexual thought was on their mind in crowded places. Because this was in the US, she carried a Taser in case of attack. One of the patients had allegedly tried to sexually attack one of the staff in the past. It probably goes without saying that people in this facility had little in common with our average celebrity with a roving eye.

In the situations she described, however, what seemed to be at work was not addiction so much as an actual difficulty understanding which actions were inappropriate. This version of hypersexuality I heard described was far different, both in type and degree, from the behaviour of most of the people claiming 'sex addiction'.

It's likely that most self-proclaimed sex addicts are not really experiencing a severe and specific sexual disorder. The people who are, are people who might be diagnosed as psychotic, sociopathic, or character-disordered. Or their inappropriate actions might be part of a larger developmental disorder, such as Prader-Willi syndrome. These people don't need to be confused with Tiger Woods having an introspective retreat and twice-daily group sessions. They need deep therapy, medication, interventions, or other intensive treatment, and a label like sex 'addiction' is simply not relevant. The same mechanism is not operating with these people as it is with someone who 'feels bad' after sex, or masturbates 'too much'.

Nymphomania has long been a term applied to women thought to have too great an interest in sex. But there is a word that was applied to an even greater proportion of the female population, and is still used as an insult even today: hysteria.

Up until the seventeenth century, hysteria referred to a condition thought to be caused by disturbances of the uterus (from the Greek *hystera* – uterus). In the second century, the Roman physician Galen described hysteria as a disease caused by sexual deprivation. Nuns, virgins, and widows were especially susceptible. Some sources as recently as the 1850s claimed 25 per cent of all women suffered from the disease; other sources list dozens of supposed symptoms of hysteria.

Women who suffered from hysteria in medieval or Renaissance periods were prescribed intercourse if married, and pelvic massage – masturbation to you and me – if single. Naturally, since touching yourself is a sin, a midwife would have to do it. Ooh er, matron! Other cures included bed rest, bland food, and sensory deprivation.

Over time, doctors became more involved in treating hysteria. The invention of massage devices became more common, with hydrotherapy devices available in Bath. By the mid-nineteenth century, such treatments were popular at bathing resorts worldwide. Wind-up vibrators were available for physician use by the 1870s.

By the twentieth century, widespread electricity brought the vibrator to the home market, and it became a popular home appliance. In fact, it was widely available years before either the electric vacuum cleaner or the electric iron. A Sears catalogue from 1918 includes a portable vibrator 'with three applicators ... very useful and satisfactory for home service'.

Because hysteria had so many potential symptoms, it was possible for any unidentifiable ailment in a woman to be called hysteria. As medical fashions changed and diagnostic techniques improved, the number of cases steadily decreased. For instance, before the introduction of electroencephalography, epilepsy was frequently confused with hysteria. Some cases that would once have been labelled hysteria were reclassified by psychiatry as anxiety or other disorders. Today, some of the more severe symptoms once attributed to hysteria fall under diagnoses such as schizophrenia, conversion disorder, and anxiety attacks.

But the idea that there is such a thing as *too little* sex continues regardless. On Patrick Carnes' website he describes a companion diagnosis to sexual addiction that he calls 'sexual anorexia'. And, what's more, a large number of small-scale, limited studies and press releases have recently been making the rounds, convincing people that there is a biological origin to this 'widespread problem'.

'Women with low libidos "have different brains"', said the *Telegraph*.[40] 'Libido problems "brain not mind"', claimed the BBC.[41] The reports were in response to a study conducted in the US claiming to demonstrate a difference between 'normal' women and those with the 'hypoactive sexual desire disorder' (HSDD) diagnosis. The BBC recently implemented a policy of linking to original research papers when reporting about science, and yet no such paper was linked in their coverage of his claim … probably because it was only a planned conference presentation, and hadn't even been written up and submitted for review.

So, what were the results? The researchers took nineteen volunteers with a clinical diagnosis of HSDD and seven with 'normal sexual function'. The women watched television for half an hour, with programming switching every minute between a blue screen, everyday programmes, and erotic videos. Brain activity was monitored by MRI (magnetic resonance imaging).

According to the press releases, 'women with normal sexual function had greater activation in superior frontal and supramarginal gyri', whereas 'women with HSDD exhibited greater activation in the inferior frontal, primary motor, and insular cortices.' But how each region of the brain relates to arousal in women is actually unknown. And as always, correlation is not causation – proving that would take far, far more work than a short-term study of twenty-six people.

As far as these things go, the amount of attention in the press seems out of proportion to what is clearly a small and prospective study. And as the only study to suggest this kind of aetiology for lack of sexual desire, surely far more needs to be done before saying for certain whether the disorder is physiological in origin – or if it even exists at all.

When it comes to diagnosing medical problems, everything we know starts with small observations. Over time, these are confirmed by larger studies, covering longer time periods, of more people. Epidemiology goes hand in hand with experimental research to help a picture start to form. With a combination of approaches, over time, scientists can start to tease out the potential causes of an identifiable problem. A single study that recruited twenty-six people? And the relationship between what was found and the criteria for subjects to be included? It's not enough.

So, just what is HSDD, and how were the afflicted volunteers diagnosed? The disorder is listed under the Sexual and Gender Identity section of the DSM-IV and was known as inhibited sexual desire disorder in earlier versions. Claims are made that it can be diagnosed using just five yes-or-no questions.

The diagnostic questions include asking whether someone is receptive to their partner's come-ons, ever loses interest in sex once it begins, and whether they feel sexual desire.

As before, there are no time parameters given on any of the questions, and no measures of frequency or severity.

If these questions seem vague, that's because they are. The DSM estimated that about 20 per cent of the population had HSDD, and with such a blunt diagnostic tool, that high number is unsurprising. And HSDD can be 'acquired', or in other words, a person might have felt desire before, but doesn't any more. With such broad criteria, and a lack of wide-scale study, it's possible any number of claims could be made about the origin of a lack of sexual desire ... but it doesn't make them proven.

Combine this with the extensive search for a 'female Viagra', and the utter failure of pharmaceutical companies to find one, and you start to wonder if HSDD even exists at all.

HSDD fits into a history of attempts to give strict guidelines to what is 'normal'. The diagnosis ignores the social factors that can influence expression of sexuality, not to mention relationship context – I would consider myself highly interested in sex, but have definitely gone off it when having relationship problems. Is that really a good basis for diagnosing a mental disorder?

While nymphomania and hysteria have fallen by the wayside as medical diagnoses, it seems we are unwilling to let go of a tendency to define what is the 'right' amount of sex. With more and more clinical interest in 'sexual addiction' and 'hypoactive sexual desire', it's hard to see how exactly things have changed.

*

Bermuda, 1961. At the nuclear arms summit, Prime Minister Harold Macmillan was mortified to discover an intern of President Kennedy's tucked in the back of a limousine, waiting to service JFK. Kennedy's excuse? Withdrawal symptoms. 'If I don't have a woman for three days, I get terrible headaches.'[42]

But do the rich and famous really have an illness, or is their behaviour more a result of opportunity?

American feminist author Gloria Steinem called President Clinton a 'sex addict' after his affair with Monica Lewinsky. 'He's sick – he's got an addiction', said former president Gerald Ford. 'He needs treatment.'[43]

This kind of judgement is pure speculation. Steinem is not a therapist, and neither is Ford. What the realities are of why he cheated on his wife, we may never know. The handful of known affairs he has had hardly seems outside the norm. Is it addiction? Are any of us actually in a position to judge that from the outside?

Jack Morin, author of *The Erotic Mind*, theorised why people with a lot to lose still engage in what seems to be – from the perspective of the viewer at home – risky behaviour. 'The adrenalin and other chemical charges pump up the excitement ... It's so common in the sex lives of everyday people that it would be a huge mistake to pathologize it. This is mainstream sexual behavior.'[44]

For these celebrities, is it an addiction at work, or simply a common desire for immediate or intense gratification? Probably most young men would struggle to turn down a sudden abundance of female attention. That much hasn't changed. What people say when they're caught out has changed.

In the past, a famous person embroiled in a sex scandal might have owned up to simple bad decisions. Take Hugh Grant, who, after the Divine Brown fiasco, went on *The Tonight Show with Jay Leno* and said, 'I think you know in life what's a good thing to do and what's a bad thing, and I did a bad thing.' Quite simply, he acknowledged that the temptation might have been difficult to resist – but that is a far cry from claiming it's impossible.

According to Dr Philip Hopley, an addiction specialist at the Priory, 'The major concern is where sex-related problem behaviour is labelled an "addiction" when in fact poor decision-making and/or impulse control lie at the root of the problem.' When people talk about what is normal, average, or healthy when it comes to sex, these are not concepts that are well defined. There are no recommended limits for adults with data to back it up as there are for alcohol. And even Patrick Carnes, the 'man who wrote the book' on sex addiction, admits that 83 per cent of currently diagnosed sex addicts have some other kind of addiction. The real problem those patients face probably goes far beyond the symptom of sex.

It seems to be that in the case of true compulsive behaviour there are other factors at work. Alcohol and drug misuse are relevant, because they can have a significant disinhibiting effect. With a number of the celebrity cases in the media, accusations of drug or alcohol misuse seem to go hand-in-hand with the sex 'addiction'.

Calling compulsive sex an addiction blames bad choices on a disease. Real, physiological addiction to alcohol and chemical substances has long been demonstrated. Making the leap from a set of well-established mental and physical maladies to something like this seems like a misuse of the term in all but a minority of cases.

Phillip Hodson from the British Association of Counselling and Psychotherapy has pointed out the differences between something we have a biological urge to pursue, like sex, and something like drugs or alcohol. Sex is hard-wired in us; having a three-martini lunch isn't. 'It's the same with eating. You cannot really be "addicted" to normal drives. What's the cure – to stop procreating or eating?'

Criticism of the 'sex addiction' industry is not new, either – but coverage of the criticism rarely makes it into the mainstream press. In 1988, it was being written in peer-reviewed journals how 'sexual addiction and sexual compulsion represent pseudoscientific codifications of prevailing erotic values rather than *bona fide* clinical categories.'[45] In other words, the diagnoses represent not real problems, but perceived problems, as defined by what society thinks is right at that particular time. But the number of people promoting the idea of widespread sex addiction continues regardless, with more than 1000 citations for the paper that first named the phenomenon – the one that claimed more than 40 per cent of people may suffer from the affliction.

The reasons for such potentially 'false epidemics' are numerous. They address societal unease with changing modes of behaviour: we know previous generations probably had less casual sex, and almost all of us had at least some religious indoctrination condemning it. They benefit a set of practitioners: people who get in early and become 'names' can add to their case studies and overall prestige. Where pharmaceutical treatments can be developed, epidemics are profitable for drug companies. And inclusion in the DSM is the gold seal: if patients' problems can be named, their psychiatric care will be paid for by insurance.

Sex addiction implies that there are limits to healthy sex that are universal. For instance, masturbation is okay, but more than once a day is suspect. Is there evidence for this seemingly arbitrary line? Anyone here ever been a teenager in the first grip of hormonal changes? The belief seems to be that sex is only healthy when it is confined and in a relationship, or sporadic and tame. It promotes an idea that the goal of sex should always be intimacy and that sex needs love to give it meaning. Enjoyment of sex for its own sake is verboten.

But remember that in the recent past, it was thought that sex needed procreation in order to have meaning. Mores of a previous age held that birth control was sinful. So perhaps this idea of sex having a meaning, as such, should be abandoned.

The idea of 'sex addiction' gives the impression that sex is inherently dangerous, that giving in to 'temptations' like pornography, masturbation, or affairs makes us 'addicted'. The model of addiction, where a single exposure is enough to tip some people into uncontrollable drinking or drug taking is applied to something that humans in general should not abstain from completely.

What we must consider is that the behaviour 'sex addicts' describe might be simply an example of compulsive behaviour, rather than a distinct illness. And we should consider how the criteria defining sexual addiction might be viewed in cultures not in the West, where relationships are regarded differently.

It may all seem very amusing to us now, looking back at the acid-swabbing and ice-bathing past, reading about bizarre treatments for things that don't exist. But we should remember that nymphomania was considered to be not only real, but also dangerous – and treatable. No doubt a number of people became very wealthy indeed diagnosing and medicalising this 'problem'.

In the mid-twentieth century, sex researcher Alfred Kinsey famously quipped that a nymphomaniac is simply 'someone who has more sex than you'. As knowledge of human sexuality advanced, the idea of the nymphomaniac became more a witty punchline than an actual phenomenon.

If good research and rational thought have taught us anything about sex, it's that being a sexual person is complex, and some people feel shame about it. Codifying people's shame about sex, however, hardly seems likely to help our understanding of healthy sexuality.

It's not a new trend: the concept of some kinds of sex as sin, and the origin of sin as sickness. Historic attempts to 'cure' homosexuality, nymphomania, and masturbation have been a far more recent part of our past than we generally admit. And those 'cures' have been pushed by therapists and scientists with gains to make just as much as by moral crusaders.

3

MYTH: Modern culture encourages early sexualisation of children, leads to more sexual activity among teens, and promotes violence against women.

It is a capital mistake to theorise before you have all the evidence. It biases the judgment. Insensibly one begins to twist facts to suit theories, instead of theories to suit facts.

Sherlock Holmes in
A Study in Scarlet by Sir Arthur Conan Doyle

One of the bestselling books of the late nineteenth century was *Plain Facts for Old and Young*, first published in 1881 with editions on the shelves until 1917. And as far as advice about young people went, this was one book that was not afraid to put its cards on the table:

The juvenile parties so common now-a-days, at which little ones of both sexes, of ages varying from four or five years to ten or twelve, with wonderful precocity and truthfulness imitate the conduct of their elders at fashionable dinners, cannot be too much deprecated.

It's hard to imagine disapproving of kids sitting at the dinner table, but the past, as they say, is another country. The rapid social changes wrought by the Industrial Revolution no doubt threw all previous mores into question, especially regarding boys and girls. After all, in the nineteenth century, what was considered 'too young' was a little different, and the age of social intercourse was not far off the age of married intercourse. Until 1929, girls as young as twelve and boys of fourteen could legally marry in Scotland without parental consent. This had also been true in England until the mid-eighteenth century.

In times past, the extended adolescence of the teenage years did not exist. People were either children, or they were adults, and that was that.

But, even accounting for the march of time, some more recent trends do give us pause for thought. The clothes available for girls these days can look surprisingly racy. Magazines and television seem to aim explicit talk at an ever younger audience. Pornography and other adult-orientated materials are not difficult to come by. That extended period between childhood and grown-up life, which flourished in society after World War II, seems increasingly encroached upon by sexual images and products.

At first glance, the worries about children and sexualisation seem to have reached a consensus. Pretty much everyone believes it causes harm – everything from low self-esteem and early sexual activity to sexual and gender-related violence. Government, news media, and an array of non-profit organisations agree. The research evidence, they claim, is staggering. Are they correct? Or does examining the issue from another perspective give us a different picture entirely?

Probably the hardest part of being a parent these days is negotiating what is appropriate in a world where much has changed.

Parents, and people in general, are rightly concerned about the effects of an increasingly consumerist society on kids. I fully support the right of parents to enforce their own standards – deciding what is and isn't appropriate is a complex balancing act. The age of the child, cultural background, and all kinds of variables can only really be appreciated on a family-by-family basis. And, importantly, there need to be better support systems to educate and inform concerned parents, so they can make the right decisions for them.

What rarely gets reported, however, is that the data around the supposed trends are very shaky. When you look at the problems most people fear – such as increased sexual activity – the evidence just isn't there. And in the few instances when people bother to talk to children, most of them actually have a more balanced and mature approach to modern culture than commentators give them credit for.

Various claims have been made around this issue. But are we being given evidence and solid policy, or assumptions, agendas, and sloppy analysis? More worryingly, is the outcome being decided without even consulting parents, educators, and children?

'Sexualisation' is a difficult concept to pin down. To some, it could mean children imitating grown women, such as the furore over Jordan letting her toddler daughter have a go at false eyelashes, or little girls dancing like Beyoncé on YouTube. To others, it could mean excessively gendered clothing, such as 'Future WAG' T-shirts and an avalanche of lurid pink. And it's easy to see how, to different people at different times, either, both, or neither of these examples might count as 'sexualisation'.

Childhood is a jealously guarded notion, not least because people associate it with innocence. And in recent years the claim that sexualisation had gone too far have only got louder and more insistent. Indeed, when Kirsty Wark waved around a padded bra for ten-year-olds on an episode of *Newsnight Review* in 2010, it seemed like sexualising material had reached full saturation.

Now, Kirsty Wark is a great presenter. But the idea of a newsreader trawling the high street in search of age-inappropriate clothing? Uh, I'm sure she has better ways of spending her time. Since when did the news media claim collective responsibility for all of the country's children?

And, as it turns out, there are many legitimate reasons why Primark might carry such items for pre-teens that were not discussed. Padded 'training bras' have existed since at least the 1950s. As well, due to complex factors, girls are developing breasts at younger ages than before and therefore buying bras. In European populations, the mean age of puberty onset in girls declined from 10.88 in 1991 to 9.86 in 2009.[46] Maybe shops are carrying those things not only because the public demands them, but because lots of girls actually need them?

Agenda Setters can be effective at outlining their view of how topics should be handled, and they often have cash and influence to spare. But the message goes nowhere without people to back it up. Enter the people whose claim to expertise supplies the quotes, studies, and numbers needed by Agenda Setters to push their vision. These are the Constellation Makers. As we'll see, Constellation Makers have been absolutely critical in helping to bolster the sexualisation hype.

When ancient cultures looked at the night sky, they saw groups of stars, just the way we do today. They drew imaginary lines between the stars to make pictures and tell stories. The pictures were what are known as constellations.

The stories behind constellations often came with moral or cautionary undertones. One popular tale was the legend of the warrior Orion, placed among the heavens after his heroic death. Another was the fate of Cassiopeia, a vain queen hung upside down in punishment for her self-obsession. But the pictures and the stories varied, depending on who was doing the looking.

One of the most easily recognisable constellations is the one called the Plough ... or, at least, it's called that if you grew up in Britain. I was raised in North America and we knew it as the Big Dipper. Ancient Greeks saw the very same constellation as the tail of a bear and they called it Ursa Major. The same collection of stars is a cart to Scandinavians, a coffin with mourners in Arabia, and a group of sages according to Hindu astronomy.

From our vantage point on Earth, the stars seem inextricably linked and for most of human history we have had no way of telling otherwise. But the stars in the Plough are actually not close together at all. It's the angle we view them from that makes them look related. In fact, they vary from between 78 to 124 light years away. And they're moving apart – in 50,000 years' time the Plough won't look as it does now at all.

Constellations are what you make when you look at something from a particular angle at a particular time. Ancient man stared at the sky so long the dots seemed to make pictures, so he joined them up. The names the constellations have been given by different cultures reflect particular preoccupations of the people naming them. But as interesting as they may be, those stories tell us nothing about the nature of the stars themselves.

Making constellations from unrelated information happens a lot. But just because things seem to be connected to each other doesn't mean they are. It could just be the angle, or the point in history, that creates the picture. Humans are hard-wired to see patterns and seek explanations but, sometimes, this tendency can lead to the wrong pictures being drawn.

When it comes to the subject of sex, the habit of making constellations is so pervasive that we take it for granted. Myths, assumptions, and preconceptions take hold even when there is rational evidence to the contrary.

Agenda Setters in governments or NGOs have ideological reasons for pushing certain points of view. But they benefit greatly from the appearance of research activity going on among Constellation Makers. Unsurprisingly, the result of evidence collected by Constellation Makers conforms with outcomes already endorsed by Agenda Setters. Teasing out who is pursuing independent enquiry versus who is bringing a whole set of assumptions to the table can be very difficult indeed.

As the concern about sexualisation has spread from society to government, new attempts have been made to address it. People want those in charge to identify real risks before deciding how to address a problem. But do the results of these fact-finding and consultation missions contain hard evidence on which solid policy could be based? Or are they a collection of constellation-like assumptions about what 'we' supposedly 'all know'?

Government already intervenes in tobacco advertising and alcohol prices, so if something is a risk to young people, then examining it is within their remit. And so, in 2009, the UK Consultation on Sexualisation of Young People was launched by then home secretary Jacqui Smith, glamour model Danielle Lloyd, and psychologist Linda Papadopoulos.

The review set its goal as seeing 'how sexualised images and messages may be affecting the development of children and young people and influencing cultural norms, and examines the evidence for a link between sexualisation and violence'. This is pretty ambitious.

But the real proof of the pudding is in the eating – in this case, how good is the report? Does it stand up to close examination of the evidence? Reports like this can influence policy as well as opinion. So, it is important to see if it is robust enough to have this much power. Or whether it's yet another constellation in disguise.

The report, released in early 2010, contains no original research. It starts by describing a world where girls who can barely walk are given high heels and Playboy tees, before entering an internet-based culture that pressures them to dress and act as sexual objects. It blames this for everything from violence to anorexia. It then moves into a summary of existing work in various topics from violence to internet usage among children.

This summary is what is known as a 'literature review'. Literature reviews are common in academia, though they are more often used as a first step before conducting research than as a stand-alone piece from which to make conclusions.

Reviews of the sexualisation of children have appeared before. One was by the American Psychological Association in 2007.[47] Australia also released a similar report in 2008.[48] These were well received at first, but the expectation was that later reports would take a fuller view of the context in which young people live. A Scottish Executive report, also released in early 2010, attempted to address some of those criticisms ... of which, more later.

The Home Office consultation authored by Papadopoulos is notable on several counts: it is very slickly produced, it provides loads of policy recommendations, and to my eyes it is notably lacking in the qualities that would make good research, for the reasons set out below.

One clue that the conclusions may not be evidence-based is to check the references cited. First, we look for appropriate numbers and types of citation. There are some things that do not require corroboration in order to be presented as true. For example, you wouldn't need a citation for the statement 'World War II happened from 1939 to 1945.' The evidence for this is huge and is known to everyone.

When statements fall outside the domain of common know-ledge, however, they should be cited. This is part of the transparency researchers aim for: readers can see the source material and where the conclusions originated. Whether to cite – is it common knowledge, or isn't it? – varies depending on the field and the audience.

Why does it vary? Well, if I was writing a paper for cancer epide-miologists and mentioned Richard Doll's work connecting smoking and lung cancer, I wouldn't reference it because most epidemiolo-gists have read it. If writing for a more general audience in a popular science book, though, I would include a reference – like this: [Doll R, Hill AB (1950). 'Smoking and carcinoma of the lung; preliminary report'. *BMJ* ii (4682): 739–48]. Even though most people know about the connection between smoking and lung cancer, they probably don't know who did that research, and might be interested in seeing for themselves.

For most of the Papadopoulos report, however, conclusions are made in absence of citations. For example: 'Sexualised self-presentation could also mean that young people are exposing them-selves to danger...' and '[I]t is widely accepted that exposure to content children are either emotionally or cognitively not mature enough for can have a negative impact.'

It's frightening stuff. And yet not one source is given for these asser-tions. There are a lot of studies quoted elsewhere – mainly studies of pornography and adults – but the conclusions reached specifically about children reference no research publications. Quite simply, this is because direct research into the effects of sexualising imagery and goods on children does not exist.

Experiments on adult reactions to sex (which the consulta-tion relies on heavily) would face significant ethical restrictions if conducted on children. They mainly consist of exposing test sub-jects to pornography, then administering a questionnaire, so you can see why the subject is hard to address. But to come to conclu-sions without even addressing this lack of source material is a huge oversight.

The Home Office report leapfrogs across research areas and years, and yet still claims to be a reflection of current media culture. But with sections analysing music videos from twenty years ago, the report not only feels – but is – outdated. Technology has moved on from the one-way model of mass communication before the internet, and citing technology antique to most of today's teenagers is irrelevant.

Perhaps most importantly, the report contains a lot of policy recommendations but very little family and community input. Especially when it comes to child welfare, any changes in national policy should be fully discussed in open forums. Government should not be producing recommendations without public input. And the policies must take into account any impact on families and young people.

Perhaps inevitably, when the Conservative and Lib Dem coalition government came into power, they also commissioned a review on sexualisation. So, how does it compare to its predecessor of less than a year earlier? Does it present the balanced approach many people hoped for?

The report from summer 2011, *Letting Children Be Children*, was authored by Reg Bailey and presents a number of recommendations about various types of media that children encounter.

Reg Bailey is head of the Mothers' Union – a Christian think-tank and charity. At least Labour pulled in Linda Papadopoulos, who is at least an academic (albeit one whose area of research interest has nothing to do with sexuality or childhood development). The commissioning of Reg Bailey does raise the question of whether there is an agenda at play.

That's as it may be. You might disagree. Now to the content of the report:

- It does not summarise any academic evidence regarding sexualisation. It refers to previous consultations, but does not make reference to criticism of these.
- It does not conduct new evidence-seeking regarding the effects of early commercialisation or sexualisation. Rather it is an exercise in gathering the opinions of parents and children.
- It does offer results of questionnaires and focus groups, and presents the questions posed to the respondents.
- It does make a number of recommendations, purportedly based on

the results of the questionnaires and focus groups; however, close examination shows that in many cases, the responses do not support the changes suggested.

On the surface, the Bailey/coalition review is a step up from the Papadopoulos/Labour review. In my view the quality of the writing is better, and it is stated throughout the recommendations that parents, ultimately, are responsible for what their children (especially younger children) are exposed to. The acknowledgement of the role families have in responding to social and commercial pressures is emphasised, and that is good.

However, I can't help but feel that these are bones being thrown to the few remaining Conservatives whose leanings are more libertarian than authoritarian. Because, by and large, the recommendations come with an implicit warning: if society does not experience material changes in the next eighteen months, government should step in.

As noted above, the report neither summarises nor attempts to address the question of what negative effect, if any, commercial and sexual imagery has on children. The only intellectually honest answer to that question is that we don't know. The report states: 'Insufficient evidence to prove conclusively there is harm to children does not mean that no harm exists.' That's a little like saying, 'Despite a lack of evidence that eating bread causes herpes, that doesn't mean it doesn't happen.' Technically true, but wildly unlikely. How much bad law is written off the back of similarly lazy assumptions?

The report also tries to summarise potential parent responses in a way that reads as at best simplistic and at worst patronising. For example: 'The world is a nasty place and children should be unsullied by it until they are mature enough to deal with it.' Not only are few parents actually likely to agree with this, it's an assailable viewpoint on many levels and a poor starting place for a supposed continuum of possible approaches.

The patronising continues throughout: '... We believe that a truly family-friendly society would ... reinforce healthy norms for adults and children alike.' Yet nowhere are these 'norms' defined, defended, or adequately outlined. And who on earth is 'we'? Added to which, in the section regarding proof of age to access internet erotica, mention of the potential usefulness of ID cards slips in – it's what some would consider an Orwellian nightmare.

The review recommends 'modest' clothing. But what is modest? I grew up in a hot, humid area next to the beach. Temperatures of 30 degrees in winter were not uncommon. As you might imagine, bathing suits were perfectly acceptable in public. Seeing a woman of any age in short shorts, a bikini top, and flip flops even when off the beach was not only unremarkable, but unlikely to strike anyone as sexual. And adopting clothing more 'modest' than shorts and a vest for little girls climbing trees in August would be tantamount to child abuse. Top-to-toe covering would have all but guaranteed heat stroke. Transplant the same style of dressing to the UK, and the context is different. It looks inappropriate. It looks sexual, even if it isn't.

Even using examples within the UK, different communities will have different standards of what is 'modest'. To some, it means to-the-knee skirts. To others, it means to the ankle. Some families consider natural hair colouring and long hair on girls to be appropriate and modest; others think girls' hair should be covered in public, however it looks. And, in almost all cases, what is meant by 'modest' only applies to girls. The tabloids can complain all they want, but not only is there no longer any one standard of appropriateness in this country, there never has been. So, where is the line drawn? And who gets to decide where it is drawn?

It's easy to lose sight of the fact that no one has defined sexualisation in a way that is agreed upon by all or even most people, and perhaps that's where we should start. After all, while most people consider pornography to have equally permeable lines, the law still has to define what does and does not fall under the consideration of obscene. So, there is a precedent for pinning down exactly what we're talking about here.

Another problem with vague terminology is how we define 'children'. Products aimed at teens and pre-teens have different content from those aimed at younger children. Well, no duh, you might be thinking, since obviously it would be patronising and insulting to expect a fourteen-year-old to enjoy the same media as a toddler.

And yet, the sexualisation discussion frequently invokes 'children' as if they're a monolithic group across the entire age spectrum, when anybody can tell you they're not. What's appropriate for a three-year-old? What's appropriate for someone ten years older? It doesn't take much imagination to see how crop tops and short skirts on different age groups send different messages, and that parents and retailers should be aware of and sensitive to that.

One thing that stands out in reading the Bailey review is that the way in which the results are interpreted is very leading. For instance, on the question of advertising in public spaces, the reviews claims that 40 per cent of parents had seen something they regarded as inappropriate or offensive.

Clearly, context is missing: the distinction between whether offensive adverts were seen once ever or every day is not made. And, of course, it would be just as easy to present the statistic the other way round, and get a different interpretation entirely: 60 per cent of parents had *not* seen anything they regarded as offensive in public advertising. Ever. That's actually rather a lot.

In other sections, where the data disagree with the interpretation in a way that can't easily be manipulated, the report takes a different tack. It presents the data *after* the relevant recommendation. For example, the recommendation that lads' mags should be removed from places children might see them comes several pages before the data showing that only 113 of 846 parents thought lads' mags were of particular concern. That's less than 15 per cent.

Of course, there is the question of how relevant these kinds of questions are to the public policy discussion. There is much talk lately of 'evidence-based' policy, but this kind of questionnaire-reporting is nothing of the kind. When it comes to anything involving numbers, it seems that people accept market research more readily than peer-reviewed science.

Remember: *producing numbers is not the same as producing evidence.* Imagine if scientists were to discard the enormous weight of evidence for evolution, simply because a survey showed 'most' people didn't agree with it! That's not evidence-based policy, it's mob rule.

That said, parents and children have been conspicuously absent from previous reviews – save the one by the Scottish Executive. You have to wonder why, and the way the Bailey/coalition report is written gives some clues. One of them might be in results like this: 'Seventy-two per cent [of parents] think the overall level of regulation for television programmes is about right.' Parents, it seems, can be off-message with the agenda … and those opinions will likely be ignored, both now and eighteen months from now.

When combing the data in this report, it is clear that as many parents resent the idea of government intrusion into their family's decisions as would potentially support it. 'Giving parents a say' does not inevitably lead to internet providers automatically blocking porn; many parents would be uncomfortable with the idea. Unfortunately, such moderating opinions of contributors to the consultation are ignored. Instead we are offered a swathe of suggestions that seem to have been crafted long before the consultation was even carried out.

So, it was to absolutely no one's surprise that in October 2011 Prime Minister David Cameron announced he would be meeting with four big internet providers to discuss schemes for limiting access to porn.

Early reports confirmed that the approach being sought was 'opt-in' – objectionable content turned off unless you ask for it and prove your age. If you're a customer with BT, Sky, Talk Talk, or Virgin, should you expect to be sending them a copy of your passport in the not-so-distant future?

Never mind that the idea of it being plausible, much less possible, to censor all offensive websites – and only those websites – is an article of faith bordering on superstition.

Interestingly, there were suggestions that the internet providers are not as on-board with Cameron and the Mothers' Union as early reports suggested. One nameless source at an ISP was quoted: 'We all want to make the internet as safe as possible, but we can't completely eliminate all risk – at least not without seriously affecting the vibrant and beneficial nature of the internet. The primary responsibility lies with the parents, who have a responsibility to supervise how their children use the internet.'[49]

I use the word 'interestingly' because you would have had to be a blind child in a deep cave with a blindfold on and your hands cut off not to detect this one coming. No one thought that maybe this co-operation could be construed as colluding in censorship? Really?

The main objections to ISP-level blocking are:

1. It will inadvertently block content that should not be blocked, such as sex education websites and medical information.
2. It may prevent access to vital resources for gay, trans, and otherwise questioning teens who find it difficult to get the support they need in their home communities.
3. It may be misused by people trying to have their competitors blocked.
4. There will be workarounds, making free access something that is available to some people and not others: a two-tier internet, if you will.

The internet needs to be a common carrier. You do not expect the Post Office to open and vet the contents of your letters. A telephone conversation should not be cut off because an automated program thinks it picked up something offensive. Treating the internet as an entity completely different to these is a fallacy.

But after such an inevitable lock-step to this point, and with so little in the way of vocal criticism from the entire country's mainstream media, it's hard for me to be surprised. This has been coming for a long time. I'm surprised at the people who are surprised. And with the state of the economy, it's equally unsurprising that the current government is trying to make porn and immigration stay above the fold. Bread and circuses, kids. Bread and circuses. Only, wasn't there a time when these circuses used to be more entertaining?

Readers of the sexualisation reviews should be asking questions throughout. The first is, does the literature show a demonstrable relationship between the availability of sexually suggestive items and violence towards girls and women? Papadopoulos in the Labour consultation says yes: 'The evidence gathered in the review suggests a clear link between consumption of sexualised images, a tendency to view women as objects and the acceptance of aggressive attitudes and behaviour as the norm.'

One saying you hear over and over in the research world is 'correlation is not causation'. It's a good rule to remember, particularly when looking at human health and behaviours. As with the constellations we give names and stories to in the night sky, the time and place in which we observe something influences whether we think they're related. Taking a different perspective may show them not to be connected at all.

What's the difference between a cause and a correlation? Put simply, when you say one action causes a result, you are saying there is a direct line between that action and the result. Cause implies that an action always results in a predictable reaction.

Correlation, on the other hand, means that the action and the outcome occur, but may not be related. The amount of reality television programming has risen dramatically since 2000; so have the application fees for marriage visas in the UK. Neither one caused the other. Happening at the same time does not imply any relationship between them.

Showing causation requires a lot more than that. A reputable report should go much deeper. One way to do so is by demonstrating the way in which an observed outcome might have happened, or the mechanism of action. Another way is by eliminating possible other factors – what researchers call *confounders* – from consideration.

For example, in the original study that showed a connection between smoking and lung cancer, there was an effort made to eliminate confounders. Risk of lung cancer could conceivably be influenced by occupation and social background, so the study focused on a population that was (at the time) relatively homogeneous: doctors. A well-designed study should always consider whether confounders exist and what they might be, so it's important to see whether this has been done.

To prove the link, there should be ways for other investigators to replicate the study and test for the same result. So, while the initial study of doctors and smoking demonstrated a clear link to lung cancer, this has been backed up by many research groups looking at all kinds of populations around the world. The result is the same everywhere: smoking causes lung cancer.

Correlations are not useless as a first step in investigating whether there *could be* a causal role. But they are the first step only. Keeping all this in mind, the saying should read, 'Correlation is not necessarily causation, but it might be – proceed with caution and look at the problem deeper.' It requires looking past a small-scale suggestion of a connection. Eliminate confounders, see if the results hold for other situations, and evaluate the evidence. If the results can't be replicated, well, the results may not have been reliable.

So, while correlation seems to suggest a link between porn and negative effects, looking more closely at the results, nagging doubts about the claims of these reports creeps in. In particular, there are sweeping conclusions made from preliminary evidence showing mixed outcomes.

One of the papers cited in the Papadopoulos report is a 2000 publication by Neil Malamuth, a prolific researcher into sexual aggression. The paper considers whether there is a causal link between adults who view pornography and sexual aggression.

Now, the difference between 'sexualising' images aimed at children and actual pornography created for adults is apparent, and using such a study as a reference in a discussion of sexualisation is suspect. When looking at how well a review makes its arguments, it's essential to ask whether the evidence being presented is not only accurate, but relevant.

But, as mentioned before, it would be almost impossible to conduct a study on the effects of sexualising images on children. You can't really do it very easily, if at all.

Judging the effects of sexualising images on children by looking at the research into pornography and adults is hard to do. Some would say impossible. However, many people believe the difference between suggestive images and pornography to be a difference of degree rather than of type. With little in the way of evidence to connect the two in this way, let's go ahead and accept that proposition and consider the 'worst-case scenario': hardcore pornography and its effects on levels of violence.

In a comprehensive review of data produced by the Malamuth research group, as well as knowledge from other studies, this simple question was raised: 'Hardcore pornography and sexual aggression:

are there reliable effects and can we understand them?'[50]

While there was some overlap in people who viewed violent pornography and violent beliefs directed at women, the conclusion was far more muted: 'We suggest that the way relatively aggressive men interpret and react to the same pornography may differ from that of nonaggressive men.' In other words, the pump is already primed in some people, and exposure enhances that tendency. But, for nonaggressive men, the very same imagery did not seem to incite negative thoughts.

When the Papadopoulos report cites Malamuth's work, the relevant context that it is a study of adults is omitted. Details from the research have been presented to imply a connection, and data showing otherwise – as well as the thoughtful, grey-area conclusion – are also ignored.

Porn and violence are not as intimately connected as is assumed by the Home Office reports. So, if porn does not have this damaging effect, how could it possibly make sense that other, less sexual and less violent things would?

One big question every parent is concerned about is whether sexually suggestive products lead to young people having sex at an earlier age. We can see what is on the market, but are these items actually 'sexualising' anyone?

One hallmark of drawing constellations is relying on anecdotes, or one-off stories. There are loads of anecdotes that claim kids are having sex earlier, dirtier, and with more people. Canadian filmmaker Sharlene Azam's documentary *Oral Sex Is the New Goodnight Kiss* features girls as young as eleven years old talking about sex parties. What shocked the filmmaker the most was that '[t]he girls are almost always from good homes, but their parents are completely unaware.'[51] The clips certainly attracted a lot of attention, and were held up in some reviews as representative not simply of the participants, but of an entire generation. But a tiny group of middle-class students is never going to be representative of the broader picture. And it's just as likely – as is often the case when a group of puberty-age kids get together – that being interviewed in a group could lead to some exaggeration of what's going on. It's not a sociological phenomenon. It's just an anecdote.

Giving a single example and drawing a conclusion does not make the assertion false – but it also does not make a universal truth. Anecdotes are fine when you're telling a story, or illustrating something you have more evidence for. It's less acceptable when making a point about life in general.

For instance, my grandfather smoked a pack of cigarettes a day and lived to a ripe old age. That is true. But does the example cancel out the barrage of medical evidence proving a link between habitual smoking and early death? No, it doesn't. If I gathered up a book's worth of old people who smoked and died from some other cause, would that be enough? It wouldn't. Just because some people do not die from smoking does not mean smoking doesn't kill.

Anecdotes like the story of my grandfather can illustrate a point. However, when they become the point – or worse, when unrelated stories are strung together to *create* a point – what we have is a constellation in the making. Great for pushing an agenda. Not so great for getting to the truth.

And while the Home Office reports are silent on the matter of the real numbers in teenage sex statistics, a number of other wide-reaching studies show the large-scale trends that are emerging.

In the US, where most of the 'raunch culture' reporting occurs, the proportion of girls having sex before the age of fifteen has hardly changed from the late 1970s to today, and has decreased among boys.[52] If access to sexualising media is correlated with an effect on age of first sexual intercourse, there are not many data to support it.

The proportion of people who have had intercourse by the age of fifteen has risen among both sexes in Britain, but remains comfortably under 15 per cent. In a study from 1980 onward, the proportion of women losing their virginity by the age of sixteen showed a rise until the 1990s, when the numbers stabilised.[53] Meanwhile, in the US, the proportion of high-school students who have had sex decreased steadily in both boys and girls from 1991 to 2007.[54] The author of the UK studies, Kaye Wellings, was quoted at a press conference as saying, 'The selection of public health messages needs to be guided by epidemiological evidence rather than by myths and moral stances.'[55] A statement those producing guidance for the government would do well to remember.

The Home Office reports from both the current and previous governments present a one-sided view that lacks the rigour we should expect in policy recommendations. As a starting point for further investigation, they might have limited merit – provided they weren't presented as an authoritative summary of all known information on the topic.

Unfortunately, that is exactly how they were presented. And the methodological faults of these particular reviews might not be so clear had the Scottish Executive not commissioned a similar report that was released in the very same month as Labour's sexualisation report.

The Scottish Executive's *External Research on Sexualised Goods Aimed at Children* was commissioned for the same reasons as the other reports: concern by the government that there were increasing levels of sexual imagery in products aimed at children, and that there might be harm caused as a result.

The study takes several approaches. First, just like in the Home Office reviews, it begins with a literature review. The key earlier studies, from the American Psychological Association and the Australian Senate, are covered along with other relevant research. As well as highlighting the main summaries in these publications it considers their drawbacks. Particular criticism is reserved for the one-dimensional nature of earlier reports. '[T]here is no indication [in the APA report] that the media might contain any positive images about human relationships, or that children might critically evaluate what they see.'

The Scottish review notes that '[s]uch accounts often present the sexualisation of children as a relatively recent development, but it is by no means a new issue.' Historical phenomena such as changing ages of consent to marry, and the evidence for prostitutes under the age of ten in early Victorian London – and the attendant concerns about childhood sexualisation – are noted. 'While the public visibility of the issue, and the terms in which it is defined, may have changed, sexualised representations of children cannot be seen merely as a consequence of contemporary consumerism.'

Three main criticisms are made of previous reviews (which could also have been applied to the recent UK reports, though they were not yet published at the time the Scottish review was written).

The first is 'a lack of consistency and clarity about the meaning of sexualisation' in other studies. The actual areas of concern are seldom defined, relying instead on assumptions to frame the debate, with many researchers using the same words to mean subtly different things.

Another problem is that 'much of the research suffers from methodological limitations that are characteristic of media effects research.' In general, media effects studies are conducted on small groups, which can bias the results but also be inapplicable to larger populations. Any laboratory study has to take that into account. It's likely that the attention subjects give things in the lab is pretty different from the attention they give in their natural surroundings – especially if they know they're going to be quizzed on it later.

Finally, and this is important, other reviews are criticised because the research 'rests on moral assumptions ... that are not adequately explained or justified'.

The problem with any study that assumes a universal standard for appropriateness is that such things are seldom universal. A viewpoint that fails to consider the past, the future, and even other groups in the present is extremely parochial, and because of this, prone to error. What is sexualising and what is not is a matter of opinion, and it's relative.

It's worth remembering that once upon not so long a time ago, young people sitting at the dinner table was frowned upon.

This forms only a small part of the Scottish Executive report, however. Bigger sections are given over to retail product assessment, and child and parent interviews. In other words, original research that goes beyond market surveys. The section on retailers sets guidelines to what products might be considered sexualising. These include products that make reference to sexual practices, ones that imitate fashion items for adults, things that emphasise particular physical attributes, and so on. Interestingly, while there may be some room to criticise the definitions of what they call 'sexualising', very little other research has been willing to state plainly what criteria it is using.

Of the thirty-two retailers, many did not seem to have sexualised items aimed towards children at all – Tesco, Debenhams, JJ Sports, Marks & Spencer among them. There were some goods in other shops that might be described as 'sexualised', some of which appear to be aimed at children, but their prevalence was limited. Of course, sexual imagery in consumer culture is widespread, and children do consume products surrounded by such imagery even if it is not aimed at them. But importantly, the research actually found very few such products specifically aimed at children available from the major online retailers and on the high street.

The report then goes on to survey responses to the products. Focus groups of parents were consulted to discuss the items as well as their feelings about sexualisation.

What's so important about asking parents and kids about their reactions to specific items? The fact that they are the people who know how these things are purchased and used in the real world. There's a difference between posing a hypothetical question, and actually having a real example to discuss. There's a lot of discussion about the meaning of Playboy T-shirts and the like in the media, but much of it is pure speculation.

There was a consensus among the parents in terms of hopes and beliefs about children's innocence. But they differed in their interpretations of what was appropriate. Girls doing 'sexy' dance moves and wearing make-up was seen by some as having no 'adult' connotations, while for others, the same activities were 'distasteful'.

A number of the parents saw similarities between their own and contemporary childhoods, about how they too had wanted to be 'grown up', and the peer pressure they had experienced. One parent noted that 'nothing's changed really'.

Ideas about what was appropriate and what was not depended as much on subtext as on the content. One mother saw Playboy products as 'grooming' girls, but didn't object to her son's poster of Jordan because Jordan was 'doing it for herself', not aiming at children, and is a 'fellow single mother'.

They did not support the kind of unsubstantiated statements made in books like *The Porning of America*[56] such as 'Bratz dolls fundamentally redefine girlhood – and make many parents feel as if porn is hunting their daughters.' The reactions of the parents were far more measured in tone. 'From an adult point of view then the Bratz doll is more overtly sexy but I don't think the kids see it that way …' And rather than banning items they thought offensive, the parents felt peer disapproval would suffice.

Much of the focus, it was agreed, was on girls. Parents tended to defend their own daughters as 'sensible', eschewing 'inappropriate' clothing. And if they did wear it, it was for reasons other than sex: 'It's not like she's about to have sex with somebody because she's wearing thongs, it's just a look,' was one typical response. They tended to feel that in context, both they and their children did understand what was appropriate and what was not.

Whether children do indeed analyse what they encounter critically – in context, and with a degree of sophistication about the media – was also considered in focus groups of young people.

Many of the reports and books concerned with childhood sexuality are aimed strictly at adults, with their adult viewpoint; it makes sense to get some first-hand information about how children actually perceive what they are exposed to.

Both the parents and children consulted in the Scottish report agreed that learning to make decisions about what was and what wasn't appropriate was part of growing up, and that parents help shape that. Children's views of potentially sexualising products were very nuanced, and some of the responses unexpected. One of the girls commented, 'I want something more grown up rather than just like Playboy Bunnies. I just thought it was a bit childish.' So, for her, the well-known symbol is associated not with being too 'adult', but actually the opposite.

Children confirmed that it was not the opposite sex they were trying to impress by wearing fashionable items but that they wanted to look a certain way for their same-sex friends. Boys in particular resisted the idea that they were impressed by girls who wear 'sexy' clothing and loads of make-up.

The kids consulted didn't want to stand out, but rather blend in. In different schools and peer groups, what was considered the norm varied. In one peer group, wearing make-up was considered unusual, while in another it was acceptable up to a point.

Young people's active role was shown in their understanding of clothing and make-up having different meanings at different times. '[S]omething that might be sexy to someone else might not be to others.' They mentioned wearing more revealing clothing, or more make-up and accessories, to parties and discussed these as a way to have fun, that the point was to enjoy themselves rather than gain sexual attention.

In several of the interviews the participants mentioned 'playing at' being older as part of growing up, when talking about themselves at a younger age. Girls trying out make-up or hairstyles and boys wearing hair gel in primary school were considered experiments in advance of secondary school. They did it to find out 'how much was too much' or how to 'get it right' before making those mistakes as a teenager. In other words, the children regarded those phases as a part of developing self-confidence and healthy sexuality.

It was considered appropriate not to display too much of the body or to attract attention through hair, make-up, and accessories, so wearing products the young people considered 'sexual' made the participants uncomfortable. One concern by the girls was the risk of appearing too much older and of having their reputations misjudged.

The Scottish Executive report is interesting because it attempts to address problems in studies like the Home Office reports. While only the result of a limited number of interviews, it is a template for how to conduct research about sexualisation that is worth building on.

Do the results of the interviews in the Scottish Executive report seem surprising? They shouldn't. A young girl wearing a short skirt does, and should, send a different signal from an adult woman wearing a short skirt. An infant without a shirt at the beach is not the same as a woman going topless. Sometimes a young girl wears make-up because she's trying to figure out how it's done. More make-up is more acceptable at parties than for every day. What's more, young people know the difference. It is when we confuse outcome with intent that we lose sight of this.

Analysis should always consider the context of the culture in which things are created. The violent and sexualised mythology of ancient Rome, for instance, was part of everyday life to them – their myths would be too shocking for most parents to tell as bedtime stories today. The things we create reflect our culture, upbringing, and assumptions. A good report should acknowledge that much.

But it doesn't always happen that way. Take one of the articles written in support of the Labour sexualisation report. 'The woman is naked – or looks like she is. Only a flesh-coloured leotard covers her body. Her long blonde hair tumbles down her back. She's in a cage, sliding her fingers provocatively in and out of her mouth.'[57]

What's being described? Not pornography, but a music video by the singer Shakira for 'She Wolf' – which happens to be about a woman longing for more passion in her marriage. It's not exactly being transmitted on CBeebies! By taking the image out of its context it's easy to apply the worst possible interpretation to a song about appropriate adult behaviour.

Context is everything, and kids are good judges of when someone has crossed the line. Imagining they have no such ability is a slippery slope that ends with all children at any age fully covered from head to toe and the presumption that all adults have the capacity to become paedophiles. It makes even less sense than imagining that watching strippers turns men into rapists. (Of which more later.)

There is a lot of conjecture about children, sexualisation, and violence. But there is no solid evidence to justify the grim and worrying pictures being pushed in virtually every media outlet of youth gone wild. Instead, responsible research shows both parents and children aware of the dangers of too much too soon. And while fashions in music, clothes, and entertainment may have changed, the pressures and concerns of childhood have not.

Really, the best solutions are often common-sense solutions. There is a danger of taking things too far. Policy should leave choices to the good sense of families and carers. And when research actually bothers to ask the parents and children what they think, that is something on which they agree.

The Scottish Executive's conclusions open the door to a re-evaluation of our assumptions about sexualised material. But whether or not this will happen is still up in the air.

In 2011, a sex education bill proposed by MP Nadine Dorries[58] passed its first reading in the Commons. To sum up, she thinks girls (and girls only) between the ages of thirteen and sixteen should be given lessons specifically on the benefits of abstinence.

Now, putting aside the problems with suggesting girls exclusively need instruction on sexual morality, let's think about this. Abstinence is fine and even good. I myself happily waited until the age of sixteen (and not very many moments longer) before having sex. The problem is, not everyone ends up abstaining, so good-quality sex ed – which is not mandatory in this country – is ideal. And let's not forget, sex ed has a lot it can offer besides just pregnancy and STI avoidance. Exploring issues around relationship preparedness, sexuality, self-confidence, and loads more can and should be part of comprehensive, well-designed SRE (sex and relationships education).

While there was a considerable amount of outrage in response to the bill from people concerned about SRE, more than a few counselled that we shouldn't worry – after all, the anti-sex, anti-abortion stance endorsed by Dorries has more in common with far-right American teen morality movements than with British sensibilities. Such a 'daft' bill couldn't possibly pass, surely? The kind of rabid conservative agenda that plays so well on the other side of the Atlantic couldn't possibly last here, could it?

Actually, the rabid right-wing agenda is already here. And if the life cycle of other government fancies such as the internet opt-in proposal is any indication, the transplant of American hyperconservatism to UK shores seems to be doing just fine.

This voguish concern about children and sexualisation is a well-trod path with a predictable outcome. Back in 1970, US president Lyndon Johnson set up a commission to examine the effects of pornography. One of its stated aims was to study '[t]he effects of such material, particularly on youth, and their relationship to crime and other antisocial conduct'.

The final report, *Report of the Commission on Obscenity and Pornography*, concluded that 'empirical investigation provided no evidence that exposure to or use of explicit sexual materials plays a significant role in the causation of social or individual harm.'

Unfortunately by the time the report was released, the US had a new president, Richard Nixon. Rather than evaluate the evidence on its objective merit, Nixon instead released a statement declaring, 'I have evaluated that report and categorically reject its morally bankrupt conclusions.'[59]

The US Senate overwhelmingly backed Nixon's statement over the facts, voting 60–5 to support the president's opinion of the findings (thirty-four senators abstained from voting). And so politics, for neither the first nor the last time in a government administration, prevailed over truth.

4

MYTH: When adult businesses move into a city, the occurrence of rape and sexual assault goes up.

It sounds like a joke from a Christmas cracker: what do Pacific islanders and lap dancing have in common?

At first glance, not a lot. The real connection started over sixty years ago, as World War II came to an end.

The islands of Melanesia, north and east of Australia, include the Solomon Islands, Papua New Guinea, Vanuatu, and Fiji. Because of the location, Melanesia was strategically important in the Pacific arena during the war. Occupation of the islands by various combatants was inevitable.

The conflict had brought millions of troops to the Pacific. Along with them came the most technologically advanced martial systems yet seen. For the Pacific islanders, it was an exciting and baffling time.

The natives of Melanesia watched the supply chain of the war machine lurch into full capacity. First Japanese and then American troops occupied their islands. Airstrips and planes brought clothes, medicine, food, and weapons in vast quantities. In a short amount of time – and from seemingly nowhere – manufactured goods were delivered in far greater volume and variety than the natives had ever known before.

Ordinarily, someone might have taken the time to explain to the Melanesians what was going on. But by the time the troops arrived, missionaries and aid workers had already been evacuated. Without anyone to explain the situation, the islanders relied on their own experience. What sort of event would have the power to direct these supplies to the islands? They logically concluded the armies obviously had the attention of some very powerful deities.

After the war, the supply flights halted. The troops who had lived on the islands disappeared. Cargo deliveries stopped turning up. So, the Melanesians did whatever it took to make the planes come back. They decided to imitate the people who had occupied their islands.

Melanesians took over the abandoned air bases, wearing head-phones carved from wood. They built new control towers and assembled life-size model planes out of straw. They dressed in the style of US soldiers and performed parade drills, all to attract the favourable outcome. These methods had, after all, already worked so well for others. Traditional religions were abandoned – the gods previously worshipped by the Melanesians had never been as generous as the ones who supplied the occupying armies.

The islanders were imitating what they saw, without realising what manufacturing and technological developments in far-away countries had caused it to occur. These imitations developed into what is known as a cargo cult.

The planes did not return. The supply lines were not revived. As time went by and nothing happened, the Melanesians stepped up their efforts. The ceremonies became more ingrained. The cults gained prominence, because if people did enough, if they believed enough, then the gods should deliver the result they were after.

The John Frum cargo cult is still active in Vanuatu today. Followers believe Frum sent the American servicemen during the war, and will return to the islands one day. Islanders organise ceremonial military marches and raise flags on 15 February, John Frum Day. Elsewhere in Vanuatu, Prince Philip is worshipped as a deity, and his followers request goods such as a Land Rover, rice, and money.

What happened in Melanesia has since become shorthand for a kind of mistake in logic made by people throughout history. Because the Melanesians had not encountered the full scale of Western technology before, and live simple lives even today, their assumptions were understandable.

However, it also happens with groups of people who have the means to know better. In particular, cargo cults can take hold when people try to replicate the look and feel of scientific research, without understanding its underpinnings. And it's rife in the kind of research produced by Constellation Makers.

For the most part, imitating successful people is something we do every day. At the same time we like to think we're savvy enough to tell the real from the counterfeit. When you walk down to the shops in your favourite team's away kit, you're imitating successful sportsmen. But no one's going to stop and ask when you were signed to the side, since most of us can tell the difference between a fan and a player. Discerning the two takes little effort.

But when confronted with things – such as statistical analysis – where the details are not as widely known, it's harder for most of us to tell the real from the fake. So, we look to trusted guides to tell us whether or not the interpretation is real. These people act as translators to the layman. Official translators might include advisors to the government; unofficial ones include people in the media, such as journalists. They may be Constellation Makers; they may not. The problem is, it's difficult to know.

Even trusted guides can be fooled by reports that, to the untrained eye, look legitimate. Such reports might use the same terminology, albeit incorrectly, or cite the right kinds of sources without properly examining the data. In the chapter on sexualisation, we saw how some papers were misinterpreted and taken completely out of context to 'prove' unrelated points.

This is even more likely to happen when talking about subjects that inspire strong emotional reactions. If the results seem like something we already assume, or fear, to be true, they are more likely to be accepted without close examination.

Respected physicist Richard Feynman was the first to coin the term 'cargo cult science'. This refers to studies that have a veneer of believability, but are missing 'a kind of scientific integrity, a principle of scientific thought'. Just as with the original cargo cults, such errors are no barrier to being widely believed.

So, what do cargo cults have to do with lap dancing? It turns out one of the most widely quoted recent studies on erotic entertainment and crime is nothing more than cargo cult social science. And because the results sound like things many people would like to believe, it is still positively reported – even years after some of its major errors were pointed out. This is the story of how to effectively debunk a constellation.

The borough of Camden in north London is a vibrant and diverse quarter of the city. From the Bloomsbury of feminist hero Virginia Woolf to the leafy expanse of Hampstead Heath, it embraces a colourful past and present. In the modern iconography of London, Camden Lock is as famous for its nightlife as Kentish Town and Chalk Farm are for their music venues. At night the area comes alive, hosting almost 2000 pubs, 130 licensed entertainment venues, and 7 lap-dancing clubs.

To the uninitiated, Spearmint Rhino may look like any of the similar clubs in the area. In fact it's been the epicentre of controversy since its opening. Not only was it one of the first establishments granted an all-nude licence in the 1990s, it also paved the way for identical clubs in London and in other cities around the UK.

Spearmint Rhino was notable not only for full nudity but also for its style. It gained a reputation for having a less seedy atmosphere than previous clubs in Soho. Comfortable leather chairs curl around customers who patronised Britain's first all-nude strip club. The topless dancers at Stringfellows were modest titillation by comparison. Spearmint Rhino's arrival signalled a new era of adult entertainment in the capital.

Customers responded by making lap dancing the talk of London. 'Table dancing has moved into the mainstream,' wrote Ben Flanagan in the *Observer*. 'The clubs, previously perceived as sleazy and hostile, are now seen as ideal venues for a corporate night out or a bit of celebrity-spotting.'

So when a 2003 study reported a 50 per cent rise in rapes in areas surrounding lap-dancing clubs, people were aghast. Even worse, the number of rapes was claimed to be three times the national average. As a statistic, it sounded shocking, but it also had the ring of truth to it. Lap dancing was as controversial as it was popular.

Rape and all sexual assaults are terrible crimes, as I and other survivors can attest. They are also, thankfully, and as this chapter will show, becoming rarer. Particular care should be taken with research in this area. Why? Because funding is hard to come by, the crime itself is not well understood, and survivors can need intensive support that varies from person to person. Sending the cavalry in one direction when the enemy is in fact somewhere else could actually harm, rather than help, victims.

One of the problems with reports like the one carried out in 2003 is that once in the news cycle, they are difficult to dislodge. It's widely thought that fact-checking in the media is more the rule than the exception. Unfortunately, however, this may not be the case. And there are a number of people – let's call them Evangelisers – who seize on any story and repeat it endlessly simply because its suits their viewpoint. In this way, something that might otherwise have been a relatively unimportant small paper becomes something of a media phenomenon. The effects multiply rapidly.

So, when news outlets all over the UK reported the results as evidence for why the UK should not give in to the creeping infestation of high-street lap-dancing chains, it looked like success for Evangelisers who closely follow issues around adult entertainment. But was the reported claim actually true? And, if not, what is the truth about lap dancing and rape?

The report that sparked the headlines, 'Lap dancing and striptease in the Borough of Camden', was produced by Lilith R&D, part of the Eaves charity. The connection of a purported 50 per cent rise in rapes to the existence of a handful of lap-dancing venues was widely reported, and continues to be. It was a result that brought a lot of attention to Lilith and to Eaves.

Eaves was founded to support homeless and vulnerable women in London.[60] The stated aim of Lilith, according to its website, is 'to eliminate all aspects of violence against women'. A very worthy ideal, and an important issue. But the intentions of the authors don't make the relationship between their stated concern (violence) and the subject of the paper (lap dancing) any more reliable than anyone else's. I consider that it raises the distinct possibility that Constellations and cargo cult science will feature strongly in their results.

The first flaw in the report is the lack of connection between the outcome (rape) and the supposed cause (lap dancing). In a robust study, you expect the researchers to show some connection between the thing being studied and the outcome being measured. Otherwise, what you have is a case of 'correlation is not the same as causation'. Just because two things happened at the same time doesn't make them related.

The complete lack of cited research about stripping causing sex crimes is unsurprising, because no such results exist. A lot of reports have claimed the two are related, but repeated studies from many fields have all failed to connect them in any real way.

But that's not the main fault in the paper. The giant red flag announcing cargo cultism is an evident unfamiliarity with calculating reliable statistics.

According to the Lilith report, rapes in Camden had been on the rise since 1999 and showed no signs of dropping. The number reported in 1999 in the borough was 72 rapes. By 2000 it was 88, 2001 had 91, and for 2002, the number of reported rapes in Camden was 96. Supposedly, the numbers spoke for themselves.

Only there's a bit of a problem with their maths. And here's where the evidence for the paper being more cargo cult than reliable research starts to show through.

If you look at only the numbers themselves, the difference from 1999 to 2002 is the difference from 72 to 96. That's a difference of 24 rapes, which is a 33 per cent increase – not the 50 per cent originally claimed. A pretty basic error in mathematics, and one that was surprisingly resistant to being corrected. It was only years later, in 2008, that the *Guardian* reported this elementary miscalculation[61] and started to include it when discussing the report.[62] The original claim of 50 per cent is still widely reported without being corrected, even in the same paper.[63]

But actually, it turns out the increase wasn't even 33 per cent. Rather than making conclusions from raw numbers, we need to calculate rates using the changes in population to make valid comparisons. Using rates, rather than raw numbers, is one useful way to distinguish real statistics from cargo cult results.

Let's look in depth at one year's change in rape statistics in Camden.

In 1999, the Metropolitan Police recorded 72 reports of rape. In 2000, the number was 88. The Met numbers are available to the public so can't be disputed. And those numbers went up. This much the Lilith report got right. But is that all there is to the story?

The problem with numbers on their own is they don't say anything about *context*. The number may rise from year to year, but if the population is going up as well, the rate might not be changing at all.

Imagine, for instance, if a paper claimed London has 1000 per cent more Chinese restaurants than it did forty years ago, but didn't report the relative populations for those years. You wouldn't think much of the numbers. Of course the raw number would have gone up – the population got a lot bigger from 1970 to 2010. Without context, the numbers don't mean very much.

When the population grows, you have to take that change into account. What you need is not just the raw number of crimes reported, but also the population of the area from one year to the next. This is used to calculate not the number of crimes, but the rate. Rate and number are two different things, but many people (even those who should know better) use them interchangeably, and this creates confusion.

You don't have to be a London native (or even a *Daily Mail* reader) to know the population is going up. It's on the rise in Camden. But is it going up enough to make the *rate* of rapes look different from the *number*? Let's see.

Whenever numbers of incidents are reported, they should be used to calculate the rate of occurrence. This gives you an estimate of how many times the crime occurred per 100,000 population. So, let's look at those rape numbers again. For the year 1999, we have 72 rapes reported in Camden and – according to National Statistics – a population of 195,700 people.

To determine how many rapes occurred per 100,000 residents, we divide the number of rapes by the total population. Then we multiply by 100,000:

$$72 \div 195{,}700 \times 100{,}000 = 36.8$$

This tells us that in 1999, there were 36.8 reported rapes for every 100,000 residents of Camden. Performing the same rate calculation for 2000, when the population was 202,800 and the number of rapes 88, gives us a rate of 43.4.

Calculating the change in rate from one year to the next gives us the percentage change, be it a rise or a fall. The change in rate from 1999 to 2000, or the change from 36.8 to 43.4, is a 17.9 per cent rise.

That is considerably different from 50 per cent. So the rate (which is what counts) of rapes in Camden did not go up by 50 per cent after the lap-dancing clubs opened. If you include the even more modest increases in 2001 and 2002, you still come up with a result that is nowhere close to the Lilith report's original claim. The combined change from 1999 to 2002 is a rate increase of 26.9 per cent – in other words, about half of what was claimed.

So, not only did the papers take six years to correct the error in the Lilith report, the media didn't even get it right the second time around. But the story doesn't end there.

Even more important than correcting the errors is trying to get things right. For example, one might try looking at the longer-term trends. Rapes might go up one year, or two, or three ... and they might fall the next. It's kind of like all the discussion around climate change: you can't tell from one year, or two, or even three what is happening on a long-term scale. There are natural fluctuations that can mask the overall trend. The more data we have to analyse, the more accurate the results. The more accurate the results, the more informed the reporting.

A problem common to dealing with small numbers is making a hasty generalisation. This is a fallacy that happens when someone makes a large conclusion based on a small sample of evidence, such as an initial result that disappears later, when more data are collected.

Here's an example of a hasty generalisation: let's say you'd never been to York before, and went there for a five-minute visit while changing trains. Let's also say that while in York you saw exactly three people – all of them with red hair. It would be a hasty generalisation to then go around saying that everyone in York is ginger. And yet, given the very small number of observations, saying so (while obviously not true) would not be a contradiction of the evidence you collected.

Small numbers are a problem in statistics, because the less information we have, the less we can reliably say about it. Dealing with this problem means having to collect more evidence where available, making pertinent comparisons, and applying more than just simple arithmetic. Reported rapes are relatively rare, so writing about rape statistics requires special attention.

Now, just because a crime is rare doesn't mean it isn't serious. Rape is extremely serious. No matter how many people are raped, it's too many. One rape in the course of a year would be a tragedy; 72 is obviously a problem.

It's also important to find out whether the rate was a one-off, or whether the rise implied in the Lilith report was sustained. So let's calculate rates, but this time for a longer timespan. We know that between 1999 and 2000 the rate of reported rapes in Camden rose. But did the trend continue? Have a look at the results:

Year	Rapes	Population	Rate per 100,000	% change
1999	72	195,700	36.8	n/a
2000	88	202,800	43.4	+17.9
2001	91	202,600	44.9	+3.5
2002	96	205,700	46.7	+3.9
2003	71	207,700	34.2	−26.8
2004	52	212,800	24.4	−28.5
2005	68	218,400	31.1	+27.4
2006	67	221,500	30.2	−2.8
2007	70	223,900	31.3	+3.4
2008	41	226,500	18.1	−42.1

The change in rates fluctuates a lot on a year-to-year basis! Surprised? Actually, that's another feature of dealing with small numbers. Because the event is uncommon, a few incidents either way have more power to change the trend. Which is why percentage change for a couple of years, even if a lot different from what was originally reported, is not a good indication of what is really happening. (Or, as I like to say, more years equals more better!)

But, without the trend, the door is left open for people to misinterpret the statistics in a way that could be sensationalist and scary. As an example, let's say there was one death due to vending machines falling over in Glasgow in one year, and then two the next. Irresponsible reporting might say, 'Vending machine deaths double in one year!' Technically, that's true – but it misses the spirit of what is really going on. It makes people think the risk of being squashed by a vending machine is going through the roof, when in fact there aren't many incidents of this kind at all ... and there might be fewer next year.

If we graph the rates, we can see if the trend is rising, falling, or staying the same. The years covered in the Lilith study are highlighted by the thick grey line:

Rapes per 100,000 in Camden, 1999–2008

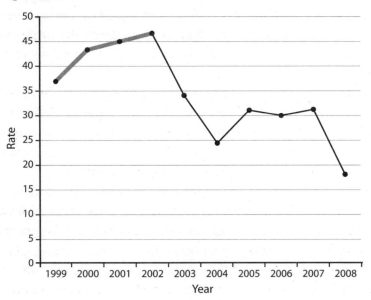

For the ten years 1999–2008, it appears the trend for rate of reported rapes in Camden is actually falling, not rising.

Another problem with the original paper is a lack of an appropriate control population, with which to compare the results. Having a control population is particularly important in assessing risk. Controls are populations where the thing you want to test – strip clubs, in the case of the Lilith report – doesn't exist, for comparison purposes.

The report makes comparisons between Camden, Westminster and Islington, all of which contain lap-dancing clubs. As far as control populations go, that's no good: you need somewhere where there are no lap-dancing clubs. Kind of like a placebo group in a medical trial.

For instance, in order to suggest a link between smoking and lung cancer, the original epidemiologists had to examine lung cancer rates not only in smokers, but also in non-smokers. You need to show that the factor being examined – smoking, or in our case, lap-dancing clubs – is the influencing factor.

The lack of a control group means that the numbers of rapes in Camden were not reported against the rape stats in an area with no lap-dancing clubs. It's perfectly possible that the trends happening in Camden were happening everywhere, regardless of whether there was lap dancing or not. It's impossible to know from the Lilith study if other parts of London were experiencing similar trends in their crime rates.

It's common sense that local problems require local solutions. What goes on in one part of London could be completely different from what is happening somewhere else. When it comes to serious topics like sexual assault, rape, and similar crimes, it's vital to recognise the factors that can vary from place to place, and over time.

So, let's run the statistics using Camden, one of the other areas the report uses that does have strip clubs, and an additional area that has none at all. Because crime can be influenced by factors such as poverty, the area should preferably be of a similar demographic profile. Then an assessment of the occurrence of rape in that area can be made, for comparison's sake. Without doing this, it's impossible to say whether any trend was locally concentrated or happening everywhere regardless of strip clubs.

Lambeth has a somewhat larger population than Camden and similar make-up in terms of ethnic origin. It contains no lap-dancing clubs at all. Islington has a somewhat smaller population than the other two boroughs and has two venues licensed for fully nude lap dancing. And since these statistics are also available for the entire country, let's throw them in too. After all, the original claim was that Camden's rape stats were *three times the national average*.

Comprehensive statistics are available for crimes reported to police throughout England and Wales, so these are straightforward to add. They also provide a useful baseline for what the national averages are.

Year	Rapes in Camden	Rate in Camden	Rapes in Lambeth	Rate in Lambeth	Rapes in Islington	Rate in Islington	Rapes in England & Wales	Rate in England & Wales
1999	72	36.8	128	48.0	75	42.7	7636	14.7
2000	88	43.4	156	57.8	94	52.8	8409	16.1
2001	91	44.9	163	59.6	72	40.1	8593	16.4
2002	96	46.7	172	63.2	109	60.5	9734	18.5
2003	71	34.2	166	61.3	135	74.4	12,295	23.3
2004	52	24.4	126	46.3	97	53.4	13,272	25.0
2005	68	31.1	146	53.2	93	50.4	14,013	26.2
2006	67	30.2	139	50.2	76	41.0	14,343	26.7
2007	70	31.3	127	45.5	89	47.6	13,774	25.5
2008	41	18.1	99	35.2	68	36.1	12,637	23.2

Now, the graph of those data. Again, the years covered by the Lilith paper for Camden are highlighted by the thick grey line:

Rapes per 100,000 in Camden, 1999–2008

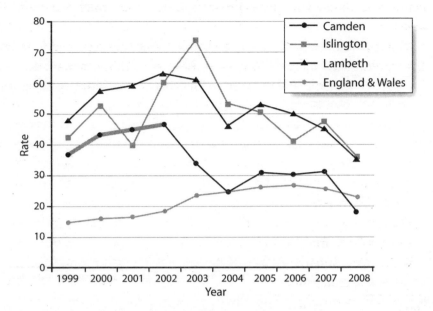

The graph shows that adding comparison changes the picture considerably. It no longer appears that lap-dancing clubs lead to an increase in rape, since boroughs with fewer or no clubs had consistently higher rates than Camden's. The data from the original study is shown to be a small blip in a larger – downward – trend.

If there was were a relationship between the number of lap-dancing clubs and the occurrence of rape, you would expect the rates of rape in Lambeth to be lowest of the three because it has no clubs. The rates in Islington would be higher because it has a couple, and Camden would have the highest rates because it has more than those other boroughs. But Camden turns out to be the lowest of the three. There does not appear to be any relationship between the number of lap-dancing clubs in a borough and the risk of rape.

Apart from the early 2000s peak, Camden's numbers are close to the overall rate for England and Wales, and are sometimes even below it. This is a far cry from the 'three times the national average' claimed by the Lilith report.

The trend for the three London boroughs shows clearly that Lambeth (with no lap dancing) and Islington (with only two clubs) both have rates that are higher than Camden's. All three have decreased over time, as well, which is why it pays to look at the longer trend rather than cherry-picking a few years.

There's a dangerous culture of assuming we know the answers before the research has even taken place. This is how cargo cult science becomes less an unusual anecdote about Pacific islanders, and more a real and relevant force in forcing policy change.

All things considered, you might wonder why the Lilith report chose to look at Camden at all. According to the introduction, it was because 'Lilith and Eaves believe that Camden's opinion and acts carry great weight with other London boroughs.' Which, if you consider that there are no references or other reasons given, doesn't make sense.

If we were to take the graph on the previous page as our only evidence, we might conclude that the risk of rape goes up not in areas where there are lap-dancing clubs, but in London, with Camden actually safer in that regard than other boroughs (and, in some years, safer than the rest of England and Wales on average). We might also be tempted to conclude that the presence of lap-dancing clubs in fact indicates a safer borough in terms of rape.

Naturally, that would be a very rash conclusion, and something a responsible statistician would be reluctant to suggest. It would require far more data from the rest of London and the entire nation before such an idea could be suggested. But that's the point – in order to make a conclusion about the effects of social phenomena in general, you need a huge amount of information to back it up. I'm not going to claim lap dancing makes places safer. My remit is to point out it categorically does not make them less safe. It could be a beneficial influence. It could also be not at all related to crime. One limited study of a crime statistic is not enough and should never be allowed to stand on its own.

Interestingly enough, though, there are other places where the opening of lap-dancing clubs does seem also to correspond with a reduction in rape and assaults. One of these is Newquay, in Cornwall.

In 2010, the paper *Newquay Voice* obtained Devon and Cornwall Constabulary's figures of sexual assaults.[64] They found that the total number of recorded sexual assaults (including rapes) in and around

Newquay peaked at 71 in 2005, the year before Newquay's first lap-dance club opened. In 2006, the year following its opening, the number fell to 51.

In 2007, when the town's second lap-dancing venue opened, the total number of recorded sexual assaults fell again to 41, then dropped to 27 in 2008 when a third lap-dancing club opened. In 2009, the number rose slightly but the total of 33 offences is still less than half the 2005 total.

Here are the incidence rate calculations (using mid-year population levels for the council of Restormel, where Newquay is located):

Year	Total population (Restormel Council)	Reported sexual assaults and rapes	Rate per 100,000
2005	100,400	71	70.7
2006	101,000	51	50.5
2007	101,900	41	40.2
2008	102,500	27	26.3
2009	103,100	33	32.0

Again, this is only a single example. To conclusively demonstrate that an increase in lap-dancing clubs corresponds with a decrease in rape and sexual assault, there would have to be many more such results, over longer time periods, from many places. However, it does reinforce the same thing the statistics from Camden show: that lap dancing definitely does not correlate with a higher occurrence of rape. And if there is no rise in rape, then it is impossible to claim that lap dancing 'causes' rape.

In fact, the question of what effect adult services have on local crime has been studied so thoroughly that there can now be studies of the studies, or what statisticians call 'meta-analysis'. A meta-analysis, or pooled analysis, combines the results of published studies by many different groups in order to arrive at an overall conclusion.

A meta-analysis examined 110 papers that claimed adult businesses increased crime rates.[65] What they found was a hotchpotch of cargo cultism. In fact, 73 per cent of the papers were records of political discussions, not actual studies. Removing these and anecdotal reports about only one crime incident, the authors were left with twenty-nine studies. In the papers that did not contain flaws, there was no correlation between any adult-oriented business and any negative effect. Of the ten most frequently cited papers, not one met the minimum standards for good research – comparable controls, sufficient time, and valid data collection. Other detailed ethnographic work also supports the conclusion that there is no direct relationship between adult entertainment and crime shown in such papers.[66]

It's because rape is such a serious crime that researchers must be at least as rigorous in their analysis as they would with other serious events. Otherwise, it's not real analysis. It's throwing numbers around without context. It's producing reports that look and feel like real research without the methodology to back them up. It is cargo cult science.

To avoid becoming cargo cult scientists, Richard Feynman said researchers must be willing to question their results, and investigate possible flaws in a theory. Researchers should pursue a level of honesty that is rare in everyday life. 'We've learned from experience that the truth will come out,' Feynman said. 'Although you may gain some temporary fame and excitement, you will not gain a good reputation as a scientist if you haven't tried to be very careful in this kind of work.'

To a layperson, cargo cult science and real science look similar on the outside in that they contain numbers and try to come to some sort of conclusion. Even if the Lilith report had managed to get its calculations correct in the first place, there still would have been plenty of clues that the look and feel of real research was only being imitated, and the content wasn't up to scratch.

When looking closely, it's pretty easy to pick out cargo cult research, because usually:

1. **It doesn't calculate a rate.** Rates are the bread and butter of incidence statistics, and a written-in-stone requirement of any report dealing with a population group. How do I know? Because I used to write papers reporting children's cancer rates. No rate = no paper. If one year's incidence is being compared to another, expect to see rates, not raw numbers.

2. **It doesn't show a long-term trend.** In the Lilith report, a small number of years were reported. Rapes before the lap-dancing clubs arrived weren't shown, so they couldn't be compared. Rapes more than two years after weren't shown, so it was impossible to see if the trend was real.

3. **It doesn't use a control group.** Control groups, when it comes to population statistics like these, are *hard*. I get it. There's no *Truman Show* bubble world kept somewhere for us to compare everything to. But, as we say where I come from, hard cheese. You make do. Mention was made in the report of other boroughs (such as Islington) that have lap-dancing clubs, but crimes in areas of London without lap-dancing clubs were not even mentioned so no comparison could be made. The rest of the country was not considered.

4. **It makes a causal connection without direct evidence for a cause, and doesn't consider other factors.** Statisticians talk about 'confounders' – the other factors that can affect your results. On the basis of a short-term miscalculated trend, a cause-and-effect relationship is claimed between lap dancing and rape. However, this does not take into account the types of rapes reported, any possible correlation with crime hotspots within the borough, or any other possible contributing factors. Again, I know from personal experience this kind of analysis can be hard. But that's no reason not to make an effort.

A pervasive feature of poor research is that it often starts from an assumed position, and any data falling outside of that position are ignored. The writers come to the study with a bias and look to find ways for the numbers to fit with their preconceived notions of what the truth should be rather than what it actually is.

We can see this on the very first page of the Lilith report with statements like 'This "fast fantasy" approach is demeaning and insulting to women ... Lap dance [is] not going away without a fight.'

It's clear from the outset that the writers of the report have a particular agenda – prohibiting adult entertainment. Which is fine, since everyone's entitled to a say in what happens in their communities.

I don't object to opinions. Think lap dancing is a sin? Great, that's fine for you. Think it's oppressing women? Great, I look forward to your paper. What gets my goat is invoking a semblance of statistical analysis. I'm a (former) statistician, yo. You're on my turf now. Everyone is entitled to an opinion and also entitled to express it. But if the writer of any scientific research were so openly biased from the beginning, there is no chance the report would be accepted by a reputable journal.

Claiming the methods of science, without buying in to the philosophy of how and why they work, is unethical. *If you don't play by the same rules, you can't use the same tools.*

The tone of the report is so attached to its assumptions that it does not address several other theoretical problems.

One of its assumptions is that exposure to adult entertainment makes rape more likely. Even if there were evidence for this, why would the rapes necessarily occur in Camden? The area containing the clubs is a small corner of a much larger borough bordering other parts of London. In addition, you might expect such a well-known entertainment venue to have customers travelling in from elsewhere in the country. There is no evidence that the crimes would necessarily be committed in Camden. Such possible confounding factors are not addressed in the study.

The paper also strongly implies that the rapes are stranger rapes. A Home Office report analysing relationships between victims and offenders notes that for rapes, strangers are the perpetrators in only 17 per cent of UK cases, and that 75 per cent of reported rapes occur either in the victim's home or in the perpetrator's. Even if lap-dancing businesses were shown to contribute to stranger rape, this alone could not explain large changes in the statistics of reported rapes overall.

In past decades, the people who have fought to raise awareness of the issues surrounding the crime of rape have held, correctly, that victim-blaming is repugnant. A person's dress and actions should in no way be considered permission for one human being to rape another.

And, indeed, this sound conclusion is the foundation of the Slut-Walk movement, a series of protests that occurred after a university police officer in Toronto suggested that to remain safe, female students should 'avoid dressing like sluts.' Connecting sexual assault directly and solely to visual stimulation is erroneous. Rape still exists even in countries where women cannot appear in public without a male family member present, or must go around covered from head to toe. It's worth repeating: seeing saucy images is not the cause of rape. There has been a long and difficult fight – a fight that continues in the name of wronged victims – to make sure everyone understands this.

So why is a group like Eaves/Lilith so keen to revive this tired, wrong stereotype? A stereotype that displaces blame for a crime away from the rapist? It's puzzling.

Such rape apologies feed off the myth that rapists have no control over temptation and are only responding to stimuli. Most people who make such arguments are not intending to defend rapists, but simply repeating things they've heard before and not fully examined. We should expect better than this from a women's charity.

Rape is widely thought to be a vastly under-reported crime. The calculations in the report don't tell us whether rapes were under-reported for the area in any particular year, nor what might cause that. What it does tell us is that the original claim made in the Lilith report – that the number of reported rapes is rising – is not true. It was not true in 2003, it continues not to be true, yet the myth that rapes rise 50 per cent after lap-dancing clubs opened in Camden is still reported, even as recently as August 2009.

The causes of rape are not well understood. If they were, it would be easier to fight them, since we would know how to apply resources. The fact that rape is such a difficult, under-reported, under-investigated, and under-prosecuted problem indicates that we really don't know all that much about its causes.

Because the numbers involved are relatively small, the fluctuations in rate could be influenced by any number of things not actually to do with rape per se. After all, the number of reports could change even when the rate of rape stays the same. There could be subtle reasons why. A sympathetic and approachable officer in a particular area, for instance. Availability of crisis support and hotlines. Changes in, or absence of, these things. It's not only hard to say – it's impossible. But one thing we can do is to try to eliminate confounders, to sieve out what does not cause rape, so as better to focus on the real job at hand.

And, of course, when you are dealing with small numbers ... sometimes a fluctuation is just a fluctuation.

Better evidence collection and better prosecution might help. But we also need to think hard about preventing rape, not just punishing it. When someone claims a cause that is not a real cause, this can derail the real struggle against violence. If the focus is on lap dancing, in spite of the fact that it has no connection with rape, it is potentially diverting resources from preventing and investigating the real causes of crime.

In addition, while the statistics used in both my calculations and the Lilith report pertain to rapes committed by anyone against anyone, the reporting when the Lilith numbers were released strictly focused on men raping women. Male-male rape is ignored in the analysis even though it does comprise a piece of the data. This is indicative of a larger set of beliefs about rape; that it is necessarily a crime of men against women. In many parts of the world, sexual assault that is not vaginal is not classified as rape, insertion of objects other than the penis don't count as rape. It's a highly gendered, highly heterosexed view. It also discounts the experiences of a significant subset of victims. If we accept that rape is a crime about power, not sex per se, then we must also expect that a member of any sex or any gender could be a victim ... or a perpetrator.

In much writing on sexual assault there seems to be a belief that rape stems from an inability of men to understand communication that is indirect; that they are unable to parse any rejection other than a firmly stated 'no'. Not only has this idea led to defendants in rape cases claiming they didn't know someone said no, it is also not supported by research.

Men and women may weigh the value of verbal and nonverbal cues differently, but show little difference in the end when categorising situations as rape.[67] For all the firmly held stereotypes, men know that no means no. Men who rape don't do so by accident; ordinary men without tendencies to rape do not do so inadvertently or because they went to a lap-dancing club.

The report focuses on the difference in rapes between 1999 and 2002. However, in its first paragraph, the report states that lap dancing 'arrived in Britain in 1997 with the opening of Secrets in Hammersmith'. So why pick and choose statistics starting two years later? If the opening of lap-dancing clubs had an impact, wouldn't you expect the impact to be evident reasonably soon afterwards?

Actually, you wouldn't – not because someone has proved that the lag time between opening a strip club and increase in rape is two years, but because no one has conclusively proved there is any link between the two at all. So, the choice of year can be completely arbitrary and it does not matter. Strip clubs are not correlated with rapes in any credible study.

While many people might be tempted to believe dodgy statistics because they sound like something that 'should' be true, the analysis shows no demonstrable link between adult entertainment and crime. The idea that adult businesses have negative fallout for communities is a myth that should be put to bed for good.

5

MYTH: Pornography objectifies women, and the industry that produces it abuses them.

Censorship is telling a man he can't have a steak just because a baby can't chew it.

Robert Heinlein,
The Man Who Sold the Moon

Which came first: porn, or objection to porn?

Sexy images have been part of human culture even before written history. The squat, cartoonish figure of the Willendorf Venus with her pendulous breasts and detailed vulva is still naughty some 25,000 years after it was carved. Greek pottery and prints from the Middle Ages aroused and amused. Edo-era Japanese woodblock prints, known as *shunga*, explicitly depicted sex in a way that titillates even today.

In some societies, explicit imagery was not considered offensive in and of itself. In others, it has been highly compartmentalised. Redefining these artefacts as potent agents of corruption, however, coincided with one of the richest archaeological finds of the Victorian era: uncovering the city of Pompeii.

The excavations of Pompeii in the 1860s revealed the extent of the Roman Empire's fascination with erotica. Penis-shaped oil lamps and figures of Priapus with his huge permanent erection featured in many

Pompeiian houses. Nineteenth-century society was unaccustomed to such frank depictions of genitalia. It was, some felt, a potential scandal. So the artefacts deemed most offensive were hidden away in the Gabinetto Segreto, or Secret Museum, in Naples so as to not corrupt women, children, and the working class. Admission was restricted solely to 'people of mature age and respected morals'.

And thus was erotica consigned to dusty rooms, considered fit only for scholars and the educated rich. They, it was felt, had the mental robustness needed to avoid being corrupted by such things. The Victorian era's oversize concern with the harm it might cause was also reflected in the Obscene Publications Act of 1857. Also known as Lord Campbell's Act, it was Britain's first law making the sale of obscene material a statutory offence.

The bill was controversial at the time, and received strong opposition from Parliament. It was passed on the assurance by the Lord Chief Justice that it was 'intended to apply exclusively to works written for the single purpose of corrupting the morals of youth and of a nature calculated to shock the common feelings of decency in any well-regulated mind'.

Prior to that period, erotic art and literature had enjoyed widespread success, particularly with the advent of cheap printing following the Renaissance. So-called 'whore dialogues', popular in the Enlightenment, were tales of naïve young girls being 'instructed' on sex by older women. They included snippets of philosophy, herbal folklore, satire, anti-clericalism, and oh yes – hot lesbian action. We'd call it pornography today, but the use of that word as a blanket term for all erotica was really a Victorian invention.

The word 'pornography' comes from Greek roots: *porno-*, related to prostitution; *graphos*, to write. Stories about hookers, in other words. But the term as we use it now did not enter the lexicon until far later. People in the nineteenth century became more worried about drawing a line between what was art and what was obscene. Those worries helped shape the view of what today is labelled 'pornography' versus what is labelled 'erotica' – even though few people, if any, can give a clear idea of the difference.

'Obscenity', meanwhile, comes from the Latin *obscenus*, meaning repulsive or detestable. Something obscene is something that is offensive to the morality of the time, something taboo. The definition of obscenity is different in different cultures, and even people in the same culture can disagree about what is obscene. Many laws have tried to define obscenity. While erotic imagery can be defined as obscene, it isn't always considered so, and some laws recognise this.

The Hicklin Test was one early attempt to distinguish between these concepts. Dating from a 1868 court case, it attempted to formally define the terms 'pornography' and 'obscenity'. Unlike Lord Campbell's Act, it extended its remit to include not only material intended to corrupt, but anything that could have that effect, regardless of intent.

It considered 'whether the tendency of the matter charged as obscenity is to deprave and corrupt those whose minds are open to such immoral influences'. These nineteenth-century precedents were especially concerned with the supposedly dangerous effects of erotica on women. The gentler sex was considered so weak-minded that even novels were dangerous. This view that women need extra protection from corruption persists even today.

You might be asking yourself, all this trouble over a bunch of fantasies? And pretty unrealistic ones at that. Most of today's erotic pictures and films resemble everyday sex as much as *Casualty* does the real workings of a hospital. It's less stories about hookers, and more soap operas with boobies. And yet pornography is a lightning rod for all kinds of accusations. In general, these can be divided into two types: concern about the effects on the viewer – like with Lord Campbell's Act and the Hicklin Test – and concern about the effects on the participants.

It is often said that porn objectifies women and promotes sexual violence. Is this true? In porn, people dress sluttier, act bolder, and definitely spend less time negotiating sex than any real-life equivalent (outside of prostitution). Porn is very different from the sexual experiences most of us have had. Because of this, it's an easy target. Most of us have never met anyone who's been in porn, making what they do ripe for speculation.

For some people, the first time they see porn can be startling. This can colour opinions of all adult films. Read any writing that criticises the adult industry, and you are likely to encounter a depiction of porn as pneumatic California girls. A look that last had its heyday in the 1990s, but has changed drastically since. Only the critics haven't noticed, because they probably haven't bothered to update their information.

These days, there is a wide variety of erotica catering to many tastes. Just because one film doesn't press your buttons doesn't make all of them terrible. Anyone who judged, say, all television shows on the basis of having once seen *Baywatch* would be mocked mercilessly in the media. But for some reason, it's okay to make these generalisations with porn.

Like a lot of things, it all comes down to personal taste. I don't happen to like beetroot. That doesn't mean that I object to other root vegetables. I'm okay with people having beets in their salads … I just don't want them in mine. Avoiding beetroot and taking a 'live and let live' stance is one thing. Pursuing the total abolition of beetroot from restaurants and supermarkets might be a little over the top.

The same is true of beetroot and *Baywatch* as porn. As it turns out there is research to show that contrary to what we may assume, the reality of porn is a lot different to how it's been portrayed, both for performers and consumers.

June 2010. Adult film actor Stephen Clancy Hill picked up a Samurai sword from the prop department at Ultima Studios and went on what was later reported as a violent rampage. By the time he jumped from a cliff to his death four days later, one man was dead, three people were injured, and the Los Angeles Police Department negotiators who spent the previous day trying to talk Hill down from the precipice were at a loss to understand what had happened to the star of *Cum Fart Tsunami 2*, or why.

Much has been assumed about how porn victimises women, but it's an open secret that inside adult film studios, it's the female performers and not the men who have the status on set. The women's pay is higher, particularly in mainstream porn, with women earning perhaps $1000 to $1500 a scene and performing in as many as twenty to thirty scenes a month. The men, by contrast, earn less than half, even as little as a tenth, per scene.

The women in porn also have more potential opportunities to get work making personal appearances. Of the men in porn, it's only a very few, such as Ron Jeremy, who have anything like a public profile sufficient to attract personal appearance fees, and he has only achieved this because he has been a reliable performer for so many years.

When you look at the men in porn, the 'woodsmen' are living props performing sex acts more suited to a Rampant Rabbit than mere mortals. And in the final product the men are cropped and edited down to faceless entities, defined solely by the size and ability of their organs.

In such an environment, it's hardly surprising Stephen Clancy Hill became so disillusioned and frustrated. 'I can see how a guy like him would live in a fantasy world where he thinks he is a ninja. He really had nothing going for himself,' said porn actress Charley Chase, who worked with Hill on *Tea Baggin' Party*. 'He's the quiet guy who finally lost it.'[68]

As a business, porn is surprisingly hard on the men. If the female stars don't turn up to the set, it's a disaster; if the men don't, it's easy to substitute any other cock. They are afforded no leeway at all. Many men think they would like to give it a go until they find out what the job actually entails. Rather than an endless supply of pleasure, it's full-on work, with stops and starts, the demands of the director taking precedence over any physical satisfaction, not to mention the need to remain consistently and predictably erect, something a lot of people can't do. Even in the age of Viagra.

For someone like Clancy Hill – Steve Driver to colleagues and aficionados – there may be bragging rights associated with being in porn, but only to those on the outside of the business. There's little else. Recently fired, on the cusp of homelessness, and with a criminal record, Hill's final act was a sad waste of life. Hardly the triumphant battle cry of a man exercising his dominion over women. Hardly what opponents of pornography would have you believe.

When it comes to the adult industry, many assume that women, not men, are at greater risk of being corrupted and used. The women in porn films are regarded as victims, damaged or abused, while the men are hardly given a second thought. When it comes to the men in gay porn, almost no concern is extended at all (apart from the occasional panic about condom use and HIV). The women in gay porn might as well not even exist. Outspoken opponents of porn such as Andrea Dworkin and Catharine MacKinnon, once on the fringes of the feminist movement, through large amounts of publicity – and a general public distaste for the topic – helped to frame the terms of the debate today. By and large, the discussion focuses exclusively on the presumed effects on female performers in heterosexual porn. What happens to the men isn't on the agenda.

Women, in fact, turn out to have the upper hand not just in pay for on-set work, but also (perhaps unexpectedly) in how they are portrayed on screen. An extensive survey of adult films measured male and female roles in porn. It looked in detail at how both men and women were depicted.[69] A total of 838 scenes from popular porn films in Australia were assessed by three separate researchers, to minimise bias. The results may just surprise you.

One of the study's main concerns was how characters were identified: do they act like real people, and are they treated that way? Reciprocity was another question: when it comes to the sex, are women pleased as often and in as many ways as the men? And, of course, violence was important: are the women victimised in the films?

The research found that, overall, women in the films talk to other characters more frequently than their male counterparts and spend more time doing it. They have more time talking to the camera, and spend longer looking at the camera. They are not only the focus, but also the central characters in the films. The men are one-dimensional by comparison.

This makes sense for films for which the presumed audience is heterosexual men. After all, with the films serving as part of their sexual fantasies, why would they want the men to be personalised? The men are there as a stand-in for themselves. It's the responses, the interaction, of the women that would be of more interest.

When it came to sexual reciprocity (orgasms, in other words), the women did less well than the men, but not altogether badly and certainly better than you might assume.

Women orgasmed less frequently than men. But that's hardly a shock since in videos the 'money shot' has more visual impact than the less physically obvious female orgasm. The causes of female orgasm in the films reflected a wide range of realistically arousing activities. Masturbation, dildo use, and oral sex accounted for the vast majority of female orgasms, almost four times more frequently than simple vaginal or anal penetration. They may be fantasy, but the fantasy proves surprisingly close to the reality of most women's sexual satisfaction.

'[T]he missionary position – which is generally agreed to provide least direct pleasure to the woman – is by far the least popular form,' the study noted, contradicting the idea that the women are in porn as objects on which sex is performed. Instead, they are active participants. 'Doggy-style sex and woman on top – both of which are generally agreed to provide more clitoral stimulation for women – are much more popular.' So, while the study shows that women have fewer orgasms than men, it also suggests that at least they are not regarded as sexual objects whose pleasure is unimportant.

Violent films are especially concerning to many people, and a lot of the debate about pornography focuses on violence almost exclusively. In this study, however, less than 2 per cent of films were found to have scenes of non-consensual aggression by men against women. The scenes – there were seven in total – varied from spanking to wrestling. Hardly the violent sadism some insist is common in adult materials.

A similar study looked at 209 scenes from US films.[70] The authors noted that in adult films 'A significant number ... had a theme of intimacy.' The research found one – only one – scene that could be characterised as 'extreme sexual deviance', that is less than 0.5 per cent of the scenes studied.

Because the majority of porn consumers are men, it caters largely to their tastes. And what do these studies show it to be representing, by and large? Not women who are passive, submissive recipients of male desire, but women who are initiating and involved. The films that strive to reflect male desire mostly do not include women who are forced or cajoled into sex, but women who pursue a variety of acts associated with female pleasure. In other words, the films portray enthusiastic partners in sexuality.

It says a lot about the difference between what some people claim men want, and what men really want to watch. There's an interesting parallel here with my former work as a call girl – by far the most frequent specific request of clients was that they wanted to go down on me. Men get off on the woman getting off.

When it comes to the porn industry itself, many people assume that directors run the show and that they are profiting from female sexuality. However, the reality is very different. Not only do porn actresses receive higher pay than their male counterparts, but what happens behind the cameras is nothing like the stereotypes.

It's interesting to note that while the directors of these films are more often men than women, they don't benefit much from the traditional method of distributing porn. It's not like Hollywood, with millionaire directors scooping the profits. The typical porn production company does not allow for distributing profits to the crew.

Adult companies give directors a single sum to make a movie. What is not spent on actors and production costs becomes the director's pay, meaning once the film is complete, the director has no financial stake in it. The result? The cheapest porn movies possible.

Recently this business model has begun to be challenged by directors and actors, and popular, well-known porn actresses. Jenna Jameson, one of the most high-profile stars of porn since the 1990s, has her own website-cum-multimedia entertainment company, ClubJenna, which produces and promotes films and other online content, with the profits staying in-house. ClubJenna's revenues in 2005 were $30 million. While it's hardly the last word in cutting-edge erotica, it helped pave the way for the wide variety of independent porn online today.

Even beyond the household-name porn stars, the internet has been a boon to the women involved. Many are now working in coalition with each other or independently to keep control of the production, sale, and distribution of films – not to mention the profits. Both male and female directors have flocked to work with companies such as Evil Angel, a distributor specialising in fly-on-the-wall 'gonzo' style films, which splits its profits with the filmmakers.

Independent online erotic sites, run by people distributing their own images to subscribing members, started early in web history. In 1995, Jen N Dave's Homepage, a website run by a couple who were also swingers, launched. They offered amateur porn made by themselves for sale to online subscribers – the site is still going today. Jen, who made her entrée into internet porn at the age of twenty, is still going as a thirty-six-year-old mother of four.

The early 2000s brought the explosion of the camming phenomenon. As the technology became more affordable, a wide variety of people leaped at the chance to make, distribute, and profit from their own porn. Today, there are countless independent porn companies, often featuring body types, types of relationships, and fetishes not common in mainstream porn.

There are a lot of cam sites run by bigger production companies, but far more are started and maintained by the models in the images themselves. There is no shortage of outspoken, self-motivated people in online erotica who have chosen to cut out the middlemen and manage their own careers.

Many people are interested in promoting a new kind of pornography. Kink.com, based in San Francisco, aims to serve sex-positive and kinky communities of every stripe, and focuses heavily on consensuality. Performers like Madison Young, who works both in mainstream and in queer porn, bring authentic desire and real female orgasms to the screen without compromising explicitness.

There are more people than ever inside the industry who actively identify themselves as feminists producing work for feminists (and anyone else) to watch: Nina Hartley, Annie Sprinkle, Candida Royalle, Tristan Taormino, and Anna Span to name but a few. And they are not puppets of misogynistic corporations or coerced by manipulative partners. Independent performers who produce and distribute their material exclusively through the internet are increasingly the norm. The personal is still political, but the politics are of equality through desire.

But really, marketing porn as 'feminist' and assessing the personal politics of the actors involved is not the point. The point is making explicit the consensual nature of performers' participation in erotic filmmaking. The point is that they are involved and in control of their careers and income, not unwitting slaves to a flesh machine. The point is that the stereotype of cigar-chomping misogynistic honchos running the show is as fictional as *Boogie Nights*.

Not only does the adult industry offer women better pay as performers, it is also changing in a way that means women are now more able to profit from their work in the long term rather than losing control of how their images are used. This is certainly a good thing regardless of how it's labelled.

Even though we can see that disapproval of adult entertainment is based more in assumptions than in reality, it's a hard attitude for some to shake off. Particularly in the far right, and feminism.

In 'Feminism, Moralism, and Pornography', Ellen Willis discusses feminists who seek to promote 'erotica' while condemning 'pornography'. More than a couple of recent high-profile feminist memoirs have done exactly this. It's kind of like the women who would go to tongue-in-cheek 'burlesque' performances, but shriek at the thought of entering a strip club. What's the difference, exactly? How is it possible to be a fan of one, and despise the other? Just a modern version of the Victorians and their Hicklin Test, if you ask me.

Willis points out that this kind of hypocrisy appeals to an idealised version of what kind of sex people *should* want rather than what *actually* sexually arouses them. In this view, vintage pin-ups = good, trashy lingerie = bad. Dita Von Teese is an artist, but the dancers in the local strip club are sad dregs of humanity. Suicide Girls? Approved. Playboy? Evil. And so on. 'In practice, attempts to sort out good erotica from bad porn inevitably comes down to "What turns me on is erotica; what turns you on is pornographic."'

Why do opponents of adult entertainment consistently disregard the evidence when it comes to pornography? It's clear the business financially benefits the women involved, and more and more erotica is produced independently. It could be because the evidence runs counter to their beliefs, not to mention their aesthetic preferences. And in the culture wars, what the middle class approves of wins every time.

Media coverage doesn't help. Many journalists don't report on the objective research. The coverage tends to be either smutty or judgemental because, let's face it, that's easier to write. And they are especially prone to the high drama of self-appointed anti-obscenity crusaders who don't even acknowledge an opposing viewpoint, much less reference or critique it in any reasoned way. What people hear in mainstream media is usually limited to studies made by people with an agenda against porn.

Examining anti-porn arguments shows that far too many rely not on what is testable and verifiable, but are based instead on the untestable and unverifiable opinions of highly biased, self-selecting interviewees.

Consider, for example, the writing of anti-porn crusader Gail Dines. Dines, who teaches women's studies at Wheelock College in the US, is a founding member of the group Stop Porn Culture. You may not have heard of her, but she's a one-woman Constellation-Making machine, and something of a phenomenal Evangeliser to boot. Using publicity and conferences to great effect, Stop Porn Culture is very successful at whipping up media frenzies that are high on emotion and worryingly thin on firm evidence.

Dines' first book, *Pornography: The Production and Consumption of Inequality*, claims to report the truth about porn, but stops far short of its goal. Conclusions about the effects of porn are virtually free of objective analysis. Rather than design a study that would pass peer review, Dines relies heavily on reporting people's 'gut feelings' in response to her 1970s-era anti-pornography material.[71]

What's wrong with gut feelings? Nothing, really. We use them all the time. Gut feelings guide our day-to-day decisions and inform our opinions. Whether you watch erotic films or not is probably the result of just such a feeling. In fact, if someone objects to porn for the simple reason that they don't like it, that's fine. It's when gut feelings are repackaged as evidence against statistically sound, peer-reviewed research that there's a problem. Dines not only opposes pornography, she also has offered herself as an expert for court cases regarding the sex industry. This is what is so problematic about her approach.

By basing work on feedback from her presentations, Dines intro- duces a lot of bias. The audience is self-selecting (and therefore biased) since no one would choose to attend who did not already have some knowledge of Dines' opinions. Dines herself admits the material is already skewed to a particular point of view. In terms of being objective, it is a little bit like showing nationalist propaganda to a BNP meeting then asking attendants on the way out how they feel about immigration.

The result is a carefully curated set of responses from people whose opinions were already decided. In many scientific contexts, this would be unpublishable. But media outlets are happy to publicise and promote this kind of work. It overshadows the rational, well-designed research showing the reality of the porn trade.

In *Pornland: How Porn Has Hijacked Our Sexuality*,[72] Dines continues in the same vein, arguing that access to adult material affects not only individuals, but relationships as well. More and more women look at porn than ever before. So whether there is an effect on partnerships is an interesting and topical question, and one that deserves good, multidisciplinary, careful examination.

However, Dines makes the case not by conducting studies on couples and their use of porn, but by 'a compelling, close reading of the imagery and narrative content of magazines, videos, and marketing materials'. She includes anecdotes about how she feels about those media (negatively, in case that wasn't immediately obvious).

Why is that a problem? Well, because having an opinion is only part of the picture. I have an opinion about porn – I like it, of course. I know loads of cool people who work in it, and I think it can be a tool for improving intimacy when you're in a relationship, and an outlet for sexual desire when you're not. But it's not enough for me just to tell you that, and it shouldn't be. Bombarding readers with my opinions isn't the same as producing solid data. People want evidence to inform their own decisions, whatever those may be, and whether they agree with mine or not.

The assumption that Dines' interpretation alone is enough is a bit patronising. After all, we're all experts on the topic of our opinions! Making conclusions this way ignores the many people actively working in the field of human sexuality research.

Elsewhere, Dines interviewed men in prison who had raped children. Every one of them was a habitual user of child pornography. This finding is presented not only as significant but also as demonstrating a cause-and-effect relationship. The suggestion is that looking at porn causes men to rape children.

The problem with Dines' interviews is that she got the 'cause' and 'effect' parts the wrong way round. This is a tactic known as the Texas sharpshooter fallacy and it's a common tactic in cargo cult research. The Texas sharpshooter fires his rounds at the side of the wall, and then goes along painting targets around where the shots landed. Surprise, surprise, he gets a bullseye every time!

Choosing a group of convicted child sex offenders, *then* finding that they had viewed child pornography is Texas sharpshooting at its finest. People convicted of a crime have viewed depictions of that crime? You don't say! Heck, I'll even go so far as to bet that people convicted of gang activity may have listened to hip hop. But it doesn't mean music causes gangs.

The Texas sharpshooter approach would be like studying lung cancer patients, discovering the vast majority had smoked, and concluding that lung cancer *causes* smoking. Dines' interviews tell us nothing about the nature either of pornography or of crimes against children. What it tells us a lot about is the interviewer's lack of understanding about how evidence works. But then, Texas sharpshooters have a much lower success rate when their target painting happens the right way round.

Evangelisers who object to porn love to talk about the money: erotica is a profitable business, and online content alone is estimated to generate $3000 every minute in sales.[73] That sure sounds like a lot. However, implying that because something is profitable, it must be bad is a strange claim to make. After all, food is also profitable. When, for example, was the last time you ate something that was completely free?

Even if you grow your own food, you probably buy seeds. From supermarkets to restaurants, our eating habits have long been for sale. An enormous international industry makes huge amounts of money from every aspect of food production and consumption. But that doesn't make our food without nutritional or enjoyment value. It doesn't make your food preferences inauthentic just because money's involved. As a society we've outsourced a lot of our food production; it doesn't mean people stop eating, or stop enjoying what they eat.

Just because erotica can be a commodity does not make it at odds with real human desire. After all, if it did not arouse, it would not sell. All the talk about the money also fails to take into account the proliferation of genuine amateur porn created and uploaded to free websites.

And as far as commodities go, well, porn is only a piece of the entire entertainment pie. While most reports emphasise how big and ubiquitous the adult industry is, most of them also fail to compare it to anything else. Take porn on the internet, for instance. On RedTube (a popular erotic video site), of the many videos available there are only 120 that have attracted over a million viewers. At first glance, that seems like a lot.

Until you compare it with non-sex videos, that is. On the enormously popular non-porn site YouTube, for the keyword 'kitten' there are over 100 videos that have over a million viewers. About 500 videos tagged 'Justin Bieber' have achieved the same status. Even Lego gets more videos with high view counts than on the entire RedTube site.[74]

Is porn everywhere? In a way, yes. But it's a small fraction of the entertainment economy, even online.

The money in adult entertainment is dwarfed by the turnover of all other entertainment. In the Premier League of English football, players have an average salary of £1.46 million each. Porn stars make about £190–£600 per film. Each of the six principal cast members of *Friends* made $1 million per episode in its final series. There has never been a porn film with a total budget of $1 million ... much less a cast budget of $6 million plus. Hugh Hefner reportedly plans to buy back Playboy, the largest adult entertainment company, in a deal worth $200 million – or about a tenth of Facebook's value.

Every time I hear someone bring up the money, I have to laugh. Because let's face facts: you can make a living in porn but it isn't exactly minting billionaires.

Critics of porn also talk about the content of the product as if that reveals how it was made. But assuming that because the actors on screen are doing one thing – a man being whipped by a dominatrix, say, or a woman engaging in group sex – that this is the relationship off screen is baffling. They're actors. They're acting.

'Pornography has a central role in actualizing this system of subordination in the contemporary West, beginning with the conditions of its production,' claimed Catharine MacKinnon.[75] Evidence she gave to support this statement? Zero. Instead she assesses the finished films and uses this as evidence of harm done during production.

There's a huge difference between porn acting and sexual reality. Using MacKinnon's logic would be like claiming Bambi Woods, star of the classic 1970s porno *Debbie Does Dallas*, actually had sex with all 928,000 residents of Dallas in 1978. Of course she didn't!

Erotica is fantasy. It is not documentary. We know this because an actress playing a submissive in one film might turn up as a happy wife in another. No one assumes regular actors are really the people they play. It would be silly to think Christian Bale really was Batman, or that Keanu Reeves is actually capable of walking through walls, but even people who should know better assume what they see in porn is literal reality.

Being concerned about how porn is made is a good idea. But it's a lot like being concerned about how your clothes are made. It's impossible to tell from looking at a T-shirt whether it was made in ethical conditions, or whether people were exploited so you could have a cheap top. A conservative long-sleeved pussy bow blouse might come from a sweatshop. A simple vest could come from a factory where everyone was treated and paid well. The appearance of the finished product is no indication of what went into it. You'd only know the conditions involved by doing your homework.

The anti-porn activists have not done their homework. According to them, '[T]oday's mainstream Internet porn is brutal and cruel, with body-punishing sex acts that debase and dehumanize women.'[76]

What's wrong with that statement? Loads. Consider Linda Lovelace, star of *Deep Throat*, the first mainstream porn hit. The film is almost prim by today's standards. It later came out that

Lovelace was coerced and abused throughout her career. Contrast that with one of today's most outspokenly self-determined stars, Sasha Grey. Grey is well known for her gonzo humiliation scenes, but her career owes nothing to pimps or abusers. There is zero indication in the content of either film to tell you which woman was abused and which woman wasn't. And as the adult film industry becomes more mainstream, women like Sasha Grey are more rule than exception.

It's impossible to know from looking at a film how the actors felt about their involvement. It's acting, after all – what's on screen is not the way the people are in real life. Hardcore scenes can have entirely willing, consenting participants. 'Vanilla' soft porn could include people who are coerced, trafficked, or abused. Making conclusions based on the plot is silly, and no way to be an informed consumer.

So, how do you go about supporting ethically produced porn? In the US, the Child Protection and Obscenity Enforcement Act of 1988 – often referred to as 2257 – requires proof of age for everyone involved. Federal inspectors can at any time launch inspections and prosecute infractions. With porn production legal and well documented, it is possible for such laws to exist. If you want to make and distribute legal films in the US, you have to comply with 2257, no exceptions. With the US an enormous consumer of DVDs and online adult content, a huge amount of material comes into the jurisdiction of these laws. And that's a good thing.

Along with 2257, it's also possible to verify that people working in porn are there willingly. There are blogs, Twitter accounts, and all sorts of media produced by porn actors. It's far from a Fairtrade kind of assurance for porn, but for those who are interested, the information is out there. Supporting small studios and solo producers through visiting their sites and buying their films goes a long way to ensuring the people you see on screen are there because they want to be.

But if the opponents got their way and all porn was illegal, there would be little incentive for filmmakers to make or keep proof of age and consent, since such evidence would be used against them as evidence of crime. As has happened so often when something like this is prohibited, the small, independent producers would inevitably give way to criminal interests. The porn business has come a long way since the days of Linda Lovelace; let's not send it back there.

Many porn critics focus exclusively on the women – or to be more specific, on the participants who are *born* women. There are many transgendered people working in adult films, sex work, and other adult entertainment. Not many anti-porn campaigners seem all that concerned about *their* histories of abuse and coercion (or lack there-of) – in spite of the statistics showing a higher incidence of job discrimination, assault, and poor sexual health outcomes in this group than among the population at large.[77] [78]

There also is not much discourse about the men in porn and their place on the totem pole, even though they earn far less than the women. (So much less that straight performers will sometimes go 'gay for pay', with better rates in male-male porn.) The assumption that if a man is 'getting some' he's 100 per cent okay with that is a huge generalisation … and surely one that the fate of Stephen Clancy Hill disproved.

Evidence suggests that while high-profile stars have blazed a trail for the women in straight porn to be increasingly independent and self-reliant, it's the men working on screen and sometimes behind the camera in those same films who are really losing out in the business. While the sad and undermotivated end of Stephen Clancy Hill might read like something out of *Boogie Nights*, it's important to remember that these are real people working in an industry whose stories are as varied and valid as the rest of human experience.

All the research and public policy in the world, however, seem to have no effect on people who already think porn is bad for women. An interesting thing about humans is that we seem hard-wired to reject anything we don't like rather than let our views be changed by hard evidence.

When humans choose sides, few of us stay open-minded to new ideas. We see the proof that we are right everywhere, whether in the area of climate change, or sports teams, or even something as apparently irrelevant and emotion-free as which bank we use.

Studies have long shown this to be the case when it comes to how people feel about pornography. A 1971 article by Louis Zurcher found that the people who support adult entertainment are demographically different from those who oppose it.[79] Age, religious background, and whether they were predominantly urban or rural all play a part. So it seems not so much a matter of personal choice as a function of personal history. It's unlikely many people would change their minds about porn no matter what the data show.

So, when research shows women are in fact not objectified, or demonstrates they can and do take control of their earnings and how their images are used, it's usually written off without discussion. This is a shame, because the debate ends up in an apples-and-oranges argument, with one side presenting reasoned evidence, and the other sticking with gut feelings and preconceived assumptions.

The idea that men copy what they see in porn is simplistic, and the notion that men copy and women don't is ridiculous. While images can affect and change us, there is no simple relationship between content and effect. Homage, parody, and humour all make use of the difference. Umberto Eco knew this. Panto actors know it too.

Context is everything. The reinforcement theory of porn viewing and sexual preferences is basically the principle of 'monkey see, monkey do'. Humans have never been that simple. If we were, maybe everyday life would be more like a sitcom.

Making adult films inaccessible is not going to change much about social stereotypes or the problems of either men or women. These existed long before mass media. As explained in the chapter on the sexualisation panic, there is a wide variety of research demonstrating no connection between porn and violence. There's little suggestion that the conclusion will change. And yet everything from domestic violence to date rape is unfairly dumped on porn's doorstep. Scapegoat, anyone?

And while many believe porn has the magical ability to make men incapable of normal sex lives with their partners, why is this not the case for vibrators? Men use porn as a stimulant for the specific goal of physical release … in much the same way as some women use sex toys. But to date, a public outcry about the proliferation of the Rampant Rabbit has yet to materialise, and no one suggests that using one makes women hate men. Funny, that.

6

MYTH: The availability of adult content on the internet is materially different from that of any other media, and more dangerous.

The next time you marvel at the powerful functionality of the web – or the next time you take its usefulness for granted – give a thought to the people and pioneers who helped bring that content to you so quickly.

Who's that then? Bill Gates? Steve Jobs? Tim Berners-Lee?

Or was it ... the adult industry?

Because as strange as it may seem, a lot of the advancements we take for granted, such as secure online payments, streaming web video, and live online chats, were all in some way improved and brought forward when they were embraced by the world of erotic entertainment.

This, in fact, is no new phenomenon. Porn has consistently embraced new media technology, be it VHS cassette players in every home or the ubiquity of DVDs. In the 1990s, *Penthouse* magazine gave away 2400-baud modems emblazoned with its logo ... an unimaginably slow and clunky way to connect to the internet now, but crucial then to help drive customers to their online chat forums.

The makers and distributors of porn didn't invent these things. And as the masses quickly came to realise all kinds of benefits from the online life, they're not even the most prolific users of the technology. That distinction is reserved for now-household names like Amazon, YouTube, and Facebook. But without the early adopters in adult entertainment, it's entirely possible we wouldn't have these things in the same way or, conceivably, at all.

Why? Well, for the very simple reason that any business venture, no matter how small, needs money to grow. There's a healthy culture of shareware, freeware, and open-source projects on the internet; few if any of them are household names. With investment and interest from the porn producers came enough money to improve products and turn new versions over faster. And if you're one of the vast majority of people who started using the internet only after commercial sites like eBay and Amazon were well established, then you have porn to thank for the sort of advancements that underpin their ease of use.

So, in a funny sort of way, without porn, the internet wouldn't be half of what we think of it now. But it's odd because there are also a lot of people out there who actually think the opposite is true: that without the internet, there would be no porn.

The discussion of how and whether online life affects the way we think, act, and interact dates back to long before the advent of widespread social media. People were paranoid about its effects back when we were still using terms such as 'cyber sex' and 'the information super-highway'.

It's been a goldmine for a certain kind of person and – dare I say it? – a certain *age* of person to believe that there is a fundamental difference between information that appears through a computer and information that is transmitted over, say, a television or radio.

While it is undeniably true that the internet affords access to an enormous variety of things at a speed that was once unimaginable, there is a point at which the discussion leaves this behind and begins to demonise the technology itself, as if the content never existed before. It is as if all the cultural commentators of a certain age have suddenly become McLuhanites, parroting the endless refrain 'the medium is the message' in page after page after grey, verbose page in the Sunday papers and on worthy 'investigative' shows.

And while perhaps there are interesting discoveries to come in the field of neurobiology that relate to the effects of two-way media (because, let's be honest, the difference between the internet and having satellite TV is that with the internet, *you* talk back to *it*), it's far too early for the critics class to make anything sensible of it yet. Of course, that has not stopped them from trying. Like all Constellation Makers, they too have to earn a living. Writing about the internet and sexuality is about the lowest-hanging fruit out there. And television and the papers seemingly can't get enough.

A common thread in almost all of the discussion of sex and sexuality is one powerful word: online. The internet, the rise of the internet, the age of the internet, its effects. When it comes to freshening old ideas and old morality, nothing is remotely as effective as invoking 'online' to make tired ideas seem new again. The evolution of the internet from super-secret security network to watershed-free media juggernaut is endlessly explored by those who know, and those who should know better. And it is blamed for nearly everything that is supposedly wrong with how we experience sex and sexuality.

Even media outlets that try to stay on the cutting edge fall foul of old assumptions and stereotypes. In an *Atlantic* magazine article focusing on the (negative, natch) effects of the internet, the author states, 'The new world of porn is revealing eternal truths about men and women.' Quite the claim. It also worries in detail about 'the unlovely aspects of male sexuality that porn depicts and legitimizes. The history of civilization would seem to show that there's no hope of eradicating those qualities; they can only be contained – and checked – by strenuously enforced norms.'[80]

This assumes two things: that only men are consumers of adult material – an easy one to disprove, had the author looked, maybe even on the internet? Also, it assumes that all men have the same desires, and that they are all deviant, or potentially so (and implies the internet is the only place deviancy can occur). In essence, pathologising male sexuality as bad and wrong. The flipside of this, the unstated assumption, is that all women's sexuality is natural and pure. Takeaway message? Men: only want kinky sexbots. Women: only want gauzy butterfly love. Much of the writing about online entertainment trades on exactly those stereotypes.

Such critics appear staggeringly uninformed about the history of porn and the internet. The *Atlantic* article claims that 'as recently as fifteen years ago', seeing threesomes in porn would require 'substantial effort' because it was only available at 'a Pussycat Theater, with its sticky floors'.

Seriously? There was internet porn in 1995, and it showed three-somes. I know because I saw it – so did most of my friends. (So too could have anyone who took *Penthouse* up on their 2400-baud modem offer.) But when the mainstream writers examining these issues for the mainstream media are neither digital natives nor fans of erotica, it's no surprise they get it wrong and rely on stereotypes instead.

Though you might hope that someone writing an article invoking 'the history of civilization' would be bothered to do their homework, you'd be wrong. It's not as if it would be a hard fact to check, after all, with the internet at our fingertips! Call me old-fashioned but I'm a firm believer in doing your research first.

Articles like these are not the only ones that get it wrong. Consider the Home Office reports on sexualisation and young people. They read like a government-produced version of middlebrow cultural cri-tique. They contain a lot of information, but not much knowledge. They rely heavily on irrelevant studies and disproven claims. They do not comment on any of the academic literature – and there's plenty – contradicting their conclusions. And they join up unrelated issues in a way that suggests imminent harm to society as a whole, in spite of data that don't and can't show that.

But one thing they have in abundance? Loads of surveys and polls featuring that magical word 'online'.

There is, for instance, a YouGov survey cited prominently in the 2010 sexualisation report. It's in the section on 'porn and violence', but the survey isn't about violence at all; it's about numbers of boys watching porn ... wait for it ... online. It claims that 58 per cent of boys have viewed pornography online, 27 per cent view it weekly, and 5 per cent every day. This is presented as *more than half of boys hooked on porn*. What the numbers actually show is more like 1 in 4, with only 1 in 20 looking at it every day. Probably more than most of us would feel comfortable with, but still. Not even close to half.

The availability of adult material, especially via the internet, is widely believed to be morally wrong and uniquely damaging. Last year, Conservative MPs started to pressure internet service providers into filtering porn: the so-called opt-in system. And unlike many pro-posals, this was one that attracted a lot of cross-party support.

HOW TO READ A SURVEY:
The truth behind the statistics.

The 2010 Home Office report on children and sexualisation relied heavily on a particular survey which has since been widely cited as 'evidence' for widespread sexualisation. What do the data really say?

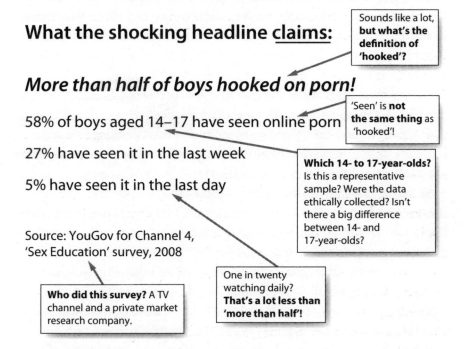

What the shocking headline <u>claims</u>:

Sounds like a lot, **but what's the definition of 'hooked'?**

More than half of boys hooked on porn!

58% of boys aged 14–17 have seen online porn

'Seen' is **not the same thing** as 'hooked'!

27% have seen it in the last week

5% have seen it in the last day

Which 14- to 17-year-olds? Is this a representative sample? Were the data ethically collected? Isn't there a big difference between 14- and 17-year-olds?

Source: YouGov for Channel 4, 'Sex Education' survey, 2008

Who did this survey? A TV channel and a private market research company.

One in twenty watching daily? **That's a lot less than 'more than half'!**

What the survey <u>should</u> say:

Only 5% of boys we asked watch porn daily, and many of them were over the age of consent.

Doesn't really sound so impressive now, does it?

On the surface it might have looked like Conservative MPs Ed Vaizey and Claire Perry were bravely spearheading the campaign, boldly taking on big business, speaking for the little people. The truth is, it wasn't their idea. The real architects of opt-in are people you've probably never heard of before, but also probably should.

With all the cross-pollination of ideas between Constellation Makers and Evangelisers pulling everyone into a debate no one seems to be seriously questioning, it's hard to see who is pulling the strings. Partly that's because Agenda Setters like others do the talking for them.

On 23 November 2010, Claire Perry, MP for Devizes, spoke in the Commons on the issue of internet porn, its purported effects on young people, and how the government should address it.[81] At around the same time, the *Sunday Times* devoted several pages and an enormous magazine feature to the same topic.[82]

What is interesting about Perry's contribution to the Commons debate and the *Sunday Times* feature are certain similarities in the information that was supplied and the conclusions made. But then, that's not altogether surprising. They were getting their information from the same source, and Evangelising the content widely.

What did Perry's claims include? Loads of non-representative statistics, for starters. One was that 60 per cent of nine- to nineteen-year-olds had found porn online. Ages nine to nineteen? That's an arbitrary and very wide range. It includes people who are over the age of consent (sixteen) as well as those old enough to appear in pornography (eighteen). But the statement gives the impression that the majority of nine-year-olds are trawling naughty websites. If Perry's vague statistic were broken down by age, it would skew – heavily – towards the older end.

Here again we see evidence of agendas being advanced on the back of bad science. We run up against the same problems with the data focusing on the internet as in so many tissue-thin studies:

1. They don't calculate a rate.
2. They don't show a long-term trend.
3. They don't use a control group.

4. They make a causal connection without direct evidence for a cause, and don't consider other factors.

Other bizarre, not-well-considered statistics making liberal use of broad age groups: one study claimed, '15 per cent of 12- to 17-years-olds have purposefully looked at x-rated material online.' Really? Funny, because you could also say that 15 per cent of 12- to 17-year-olds actually *are* 17. Stating that a large percentage of people over the age of consent may be looking at porn gives rather a different impression from implying that a bunch of twelve-year-olds are doing it.

And from the same study, the inexplicable use of vague definitions: '70 per cent of 15- to 17-year-old internet users accidentally view pornography "very" or "somewhat" often.' What's 'very'? What's 'somewhat'? I suspect what counts as 'very often' varies from person to person, but none of us will be any the wiser, since the report doesn't go into this.[83]

In what is now a depressingly predictable aside, that particular paper was produced by a company – not a healthcare or academic institution, not even a charity – whose recruitment policies involve online questionnaires deployed by market research groups with shopping gift card incentives for participants.[84]

Perry also claimed: 'A third of our British 10-year-olds have viewed pornography on the internet,' which would certainly be worrying if it were true. The figure is from *Psychologies* magazine's 'Put Porn in Its Place' campaign.[85] The name alone suggests the conclusion was probably written well before the data were collected. Despite its name, *Psychologies* is not a peer-reviewed academic journal, but a mass-market magazine rather like *GQ* or *Cosmo*. The summary articles were written by Decca Aitkenhead, a travel writer and lifestyle commentator, not a researcher nor even a science journalist.

The poll in question contains two significant problems. First, the data were collected from a single year of boys at a single school in London. Such a small and concentrated population is hardly representative of British children in general.

Secondly, the poll was not of ten-year-olds and their habits. Rather, it was of sixteen-year-olds and their *recollections* of the first age at which they saw porn. See the crucial difference? Any study that relies on such a significant gap is likely to be riddled with errors. It should acknowledge this. It doesn't.

Comprehensive criticism of the data would also take note of the fact that no mention is made of how subjects were recruited, and whether their parents were informed. After all, academic research would have to refer to this, to ensure required ethical standards were being met. In short, it's not a credible or reliable figure. But this is small fry compared to the study's greater flaws.

Claire Perry's comments came one day after an event she attended at the Houses of Parliament, 'The Harm that Pornography Does: Its Effects on Adults and Children and the Need for Regulatory Reform'. The event was organised by Safermedia, whose co-chair, Miranda Suit, quotes a particular report also cited in the *Sunday Times Magazine* feature. The article prominently mentions 'new research into the social costs of pornography from the Witherspoon Institute in America'.

No mention is made of the group's purpose, their previous work, or even any of their members. It's unlikely many of the *Sunday Times* readers will even have heard of them. Just who are the Witherspoon Institute, anyway? Their website makes much of the group's namesake, a Scottish Calvinist minister and signer of the Declaration of Independence. However, the institute does not obviously appear to be either directly endorsed or funded by Witherspoon's family.

Looking deeper, the 'research' turns out to be *The Social Costs of Pornography: A Collection of Papers.*[86] It includes contributions from such notables as Patrick Fagan from the Family Research Council, a far-right American lobbying organisation. Fagan also works with the Heritage Foundation. For those unfamiliar with the minutiae of American think-tanks, the Heritage Foundation were considered the architects of the Reagan administration's covert Cold War operations, and were active supporters of George W Bush's international policy. Fagan's other recent papers mentioned on the Witherspoon site include 'Virgins Make the Best Valentines' and 'Why Congress Should Ignore Radical Feminist Opposition to Marriage'.

If the needle on your Agenda Setter detection meter isn't going off the charts, it should be. The agenda here is very, very clear.

The Social Costs of Pornography reads as if it had decided the outcome before assessing the evidence – a research no-no in responsible circles. But it also admits that the evidence for porn causing harm as such is thin on the ground. 'The few statistics available about the use of pornography by children and adolescents are even more difficult to assess than those concerning adults ... Nevertheless, there can be no doubt that children and adolescents are far more exposed to pornography via the internet than they ever have been before.' How is it possible to make such sweeping conclusions when there are no data to prove it?

What the report does offer is a hotchpotch of statistics, some of which are at least ten years old. It then reflects again: 'But is there evidence that this exposure is harmful to children? For some people, no more evidence is needed.' This in spite of failing to show or imply the existence of a single study showing a cause-and-effect relationship between viewing pornography and harm. You'll excuse me for thinking *a lot more* evidence is needed!

It continues, 'However, even sceptics could not deny the evidence of harmfulness that is emerging in clinical settings.' Actually, yes, they would. A sceptic would point out that unless you have presented evidence, you cannot subsequently claim the evidence exists. You can't admit the evidence doesn't exist and then claim no more evidence is needed. You can't. It's logically impossible. It bends space-time and makes the Baby Jesus weep.

The *Sunday Times* coverage of young people and their online habits tried ever so hard to be up to date. It went on about the 'new' evidence in the Witherspoon report. It was even illustrated with a photo of porn star Jenna Jameson. Unfortunately, they chose a photo of Jenna that's ten years old. How up to date is that? (I know this because I watch loads of porn, by the way. Her look has changed a lot in that time.)

So, one must ask whether any of the source material from the Witherspoon report is, as claimed in the *Sunday Times*, 'new'. It isn't. The report is riddled with anachronisms worthy of Shakespeare's *Julius Caesar*. For instance, 'Many people first encounter pornography on television in a hotel room,' is one observation. Which the eagle-eyed will note is neither an internet phenomenon, nor a recent one, nor likely to be true for young people born after, say, the 1970s. In terms of pop culture, it's about as relevant as citing Calvin Klein adverts ...

which the *Sunday Times* piece does on its very first page.

Close examination of the Witherspoon report makes its aim clear: 'Political leaders should use the bully pulpit'. Celebrities, too, are urged to apply pressure. And finally, the Witherspoon report returns to the necessary admission that the data do not support its cause: 'Some of the most important parts of our laws could not be justified if they had to hinge on a proof of material injuries.'

The thought of policy being created off the back of this kind of publication shows how out of touch the politicians are. Special interests appear to be lobbying and organising meetings for them, and all but writing the Hansard themselves.

Like many think-tanks, Witherspoon has a strong bias. They also admit – repeatedly – that the evidence is insubstantial. Are they a good source of information for journalists? For policy makers? Are the people who hope Perry and Vaizey will do right by young people at all concerned how this looks? Because it looks like UK policy is being spoon-fed to the current government by some of America's most extreme social conservatives.

Many sources keep the focus of the discussion consistently on people's fears about what might happen in some dystopian sci-fi future, rather than looking at data about what does happen in our world right now. Partly, this fulfils a certain unease people seem to have with new technology.

But there are reliable studies that contradict any connection between porn and violence. 'There's absolutely no evidence that pornography does anything negative,' says Milton Diamond, a professor at the University of Hawaii in a recent interview in *Scientific American*.[87] 'It's a moral issue, not a factual issue.'

A number of studies by Aleksandar Štulhofer at the University of Zagreb have examined sexual compulsivity. One of them surveyed 650 men about pornography and their sex lives.[88] Results showed that viewers of mainstream pornography were just as sexually satisfied as non-users. Both groups reported the same levels of intimacy in their relationships. They even shared the same range of sexual experiences.

Regular pornography use does not seem to encourage sexism. In 2007, a survey on sexist tendencies was included in mail-order porn deliveries sent out across Australia. Responses from 1023 people showed that the amount of pornography they consumed was not correlated with negative attitudes towards women. Other factors, such as level of education and political tendencies, were more indicative of whether someone was sexist.[89]

Simon-Louis Lajeunesse is a professor at the University of Montreal who attempted to design a study of the impact of pornography on the sexuality of men, and how it shapes their perception of men and women. In a prospective study of twenty students, Lajeunesse found most of the men questioned sought out porn by the age of ten, when they become sexually curious. He also found they quickly discarded what they didn't like and things they found offensive. As adults, they looked for content that was compatible with their sex preferences.[90]

All of Lajeunesse's subjects supported gender equality and felt victimised by criticism of pornography. 'Pornography hasn't changed their perception of women or their relationship, which they all want as harmonious and fulfilling as possible,' says Lajeunesse. His subjects reiterated that they wanted real women, not fantasy women. And watching porn did not change their tastes or relationship goals in any significant way. 'If pornography had the impact that many claim it has, you would just have to show heterosexual films to a homosexual to change his sexual orientation.' His interesting observations, however, never fully developed as a research project, since he was unable to find control subjects: young men who had not seen any porn.

Perhaps the most serious accusation is that pornography inspires sexual assaults. But not only do rape statistics suggest otherwise, some experts believe the consumption of pornography may actually offer a safe outlet for deviant sexual desires.

Rates of rapes and sexual assault in the US are at their lowest levels since the 1960s. The same is true for countries such as Japan, China, and Denmark, which once heavily restricted porn access. In the past forty years, as porn has become more prevalent, rape statistics have fallen. Studies show that in the US the introduction of internet access corresponded with a decrease in rape (and no effect on other violent crimes). A 10 per cent increase in online access corresponded with a 7.3 per cent decrease in reported rapes.[91] States slowest to adopt internet technology experienced a 53 per cent increase in rape incidence, whereas the states with the most access experienced a 27 per cent drop in the number of reported rapes. And the effects remain even when taking into account confounders such as alcohol use, law enforcement, income, employment, and population density.[92]

There's an interesting similarity between such results and research into violence. When a violent film is released at the cinema, crime rates – surprisingly enough – go *down*. Apparently movie violence doesn't increase real-life violence after all. The theory is that people disposed to violence like watching violent films, and given the choice between the latest shoot-'em-up thriller and going out to commit crime, plump for the popcorn option.[93]

What's more, work in the 1960s showed sexual criminals tend to be exposed to pornographic materials at a later age than non-criminals. In 1992, Richard Green of Imperial College wrote how patients in a sex offenders' clinic cited pornography as a tool to keep desires within the confines of their imagination.[94] Pornography seems to be protective, perhaps because exposure correlates with lower levels of sexual repression, a potential rape risk factor.

Does this prove that, in fact, internet access and violent films actually reduce rape and violent crime? No, not really. Not yet. There would have to be a lot more research – from many more angles – to even begin to support such a claim. Again, correlation is not causation.

Loads of people claim that porn incites violence. The data do not support these claims. Porn's gone up, rape's fallen. And as the internet has increased access to erotic material, the effect has not only been enhanced, but measurable. So either they're related but in the opposite way to how people previously expected, or they're not actually related at all. Either way, it's a far better outcome than anyone could have predicted.

There is a shadowy other in the discussion about online lives. That is the availability not only of mainstream erotica, but also the spectre of material that is illegal with good reason. It raises the question of who might access such material, and whether this results in violence against other people.

Just to make clear, I'm not even going to entertain the ridiculous notion that 'all' or even 'most' porn is violent. That slippery slope argument is best left to people who just want to ban all adult entertainment anyway. What I'm talking about is material depicting violent crimes: actual murders, actual rapes.

The 2003 murder of Jane Longhurst, a teacher who was raped and strangled by an acquaintance, sparked controversy about the nature of violent pornography. Her killer, Graham Coutts, admitted to watching a considerable amount of porn around the time that he killed Miss Longhurst. At the trial it was strongly implied that pornography was not only an arousal to Coutts, but also what drove him to kill. In other words, watching porn was the slippery slope that ended in murder. That he might have murdered even without porn did not seem to be considered. The fact that he had a strangulation fetish for a number of years before he started accessing the porn in question also throws doubt on this assumption.

Just to reiterate, the rape and murder of a young woman is a terrible crime. On that everyone is agreed. But I would also go so far as to say let's not let a murderer off the hook by claiming, 'It was porn that made him do it.' What a weak and mealy-mouthed defence. He's a monster, end of. Anything else is relieving him of his responsibility for the death of a human being.

Following a campaign by Ms Longhurst's mother, a Home Office consultation took place. The majority (63 per cent) of groups and members of the public who replied to the consultation saw no need to strengthen existing laws regarding porn. A new law was made anyway – Section 63 of the Criminal Justice and Immigration Act 2008. This was in spite of the fact that there is almost no evidence to back the claim that exposure to pornography alone provokes violence.

Let's take a different example. In late October 2011, Dutch engineer Vincent Tabak was convicted of murder by strangulation of Jo Yeates in Bristol. After the verdict was recorded, it emerged that the prosecution had tried to enter evidence that Tabak subscribed to domination porn sites and had visited sex workers in the past.

The judge on the case ruled this as inadmissible and potentially prejudicial; as a result, it was not considered by the jury when coming to their verdict.

So, in spite of the fact that Tabak – who had admitted manslaughter – was convicted of murder, the papers had a field day. Since obviously his use of pornography must have inspired the killing, right?

Erm, no. There is still no causal connection between porn and murder. Just because someone used porn, and then killed someone, it does not follow that the porn caused the crime. Let's remember, the vast majority of porn users are not violent and do not commit murder. Trying to claim otherwise, as the papers tried to do? Texas sharpshooter syndrome at its finest.

There is no evidence connecting porn with incitement to violence or murder in people who are not already inclined to violence or murder. If there was any such connection, surely the prosecution would have dug up a credible expert witness to bolster that assumption. Or maybe they would have presented generally accepted academic proof of a connection. They didn't. One can only speculate why they didn't, but it's not hard to imagine that's because no such expert or proof exists.

As unpleasant as violent pornography may be to most people, it is not in any way common sense to assume that those watching it want to participate. We all fantasise about things we would never do in real life. Some fantasies are innocent, some less so. It's human nature. We must be held responsible for our actions, not our thoughts.

The content of edgy porn is proscribed in other ways as well. In January 2012, Michael Peacock stood trial for distributing allegedly 'obscene' DVDs, containing scenes of men fisting each other, urination, and bondage. The rather delicious irony is that not only are such acts relatively common in the 'kinky' community (I've even written about all of them), they're perfectly legal for consenting adults to participate in and watch in person. The outcome of the trial was therefore important, because if the material Peacock is alleged to have distributed was judged 'not obscene', porn produced and sold in the UK will theoretically be free to contain scenes of fisting and urination.

The Obscene Publications Act 1959, under which Peacock was prosecuted, aims to judge content on whether it is liable to 'deprave and corrupt'. One of the interesting things about the interpretation of this law is that while it isn't written to single out sex acts specifically, the acts considered to be prosecutable under the Obscene Publications Act are all of a sexual nature. So, for instance, you might consider images of a man being beaten and shot to be obscene if published in a newspaper; yet this happens with some frequency and the law is not invoked against it. Watching jumpy video of Gaddafi's last moments is fine; consensual watersports is not.

Rather wonderfully, the jury came back with a verdict of not guilty, unanimously, on all counts after about a tea-break's worth of deliberation.

For those who value personal liberty, it was a win. It also revealed a lot about the state of how the public views sex today. It's that perhaps we are finally beginning to become comfortable with the idea of consent, the notion that one does not have to practise a particular sexual kink or orientation to not condemn it, and that people who approach an escort who goes by the handle 'Sleazy Michael' and rent or buy DVDs from him are possibly, just possibly, not being blindsided by the nature of their content.

It was only after the trial began that I realised the defendant, Michael Peacock, was someone I know. In my opinion he is a nice person who is genuinely enthusiastic about his work and his clients. In short, the best kind of escort. A really top bloke. And brave too. The thought that he corrupts or defiles anyone who doesn't want said treatment is frankly ridiculous.

But the notions that led to this trial even happening are part of a line of thinking that is all too pervasive when it comes to sex. The sexualisation debate for example is entirely built on the erroneous assumption that if suggestive material wasn't available, young people would never become curious about sex. The idea that sex (and especially sex where commerce is involved) is unique, and uniquely corrupting, is an unfortunate leitmotif in public discourse. In such an atmosphere, someone who distributes images of *consenting adults engaging in perfectly legal acts* is targeted simply because it is Big Bad Sex.

There's a strong element of 'what's sauce for the goose is sauce for the gander' about the not guilty verdict. After all, no one was disputing the legality of consenting to being fisted or punched in the balls. It was more the question of who might see it happening. The history of pornography is littered with such arbitrary divides between who is assumed to be corruptible and who is not. Private galleries of Pompeian icons of Priapus and his giant penis were once fine for men of a certain class, but not suitable to be seen by the general adult public.

The case against Michael Peacock was in many ways trying to affirm the same arbitrary standard: this is suitable for some but not for others. In this case, the medium is what enforces the class divide. It's perfectly okay for those who, in the privacy of their own homes, can afford it. Let's not mince words; we all know the rich and powerful can and do indulge their kinky desires and would like to continue to do so in private. What the prosecution alleged is that it's not okay for the plebs to be looking at cheap DVDs or (presumably) downloads.

The bottom line is that whatever movies we watch, books we read, or music we listen to should not be used to infer criminal guilt. No matter how offensive it is. Misattributing the outcome of a young woman's murder to a man's viewing of porn might also be seen as somehow taking away his responsibility for the killing, which would be abhorrent. The judge made the right call, and Tabak was convicted of murder on a case that was strong enough on its own. It didn't need a prop of junk data and prejudicial assumptions. Surely that is real justice for Jo Yeates.

There's a lack of real courage in the inability of the government to admit its consultations on issues about sex, erotica, and sexuality are unfit for purpose. They propose easy solutions to difficult problems. And criminals jump to endorse state-approved easy answers rather than face their own depravity.

Consider serial murderer Ted Bundy, an attractive smooth talker who murdered scores of students in Florida in the 1970s. He claimed a porn addiction made him do it, and his observations were repeated and reported as if gospel truth. Respected sex therapist Dr Marty Klein summarises the problems with this beautifully. 'If convicted mass murderer Ted Bundy had said that watching Bill Cosby reruns motivated his awful crimes, he would have been dismissed as a deranged sociopath.'[95] Why give his porn claims any weight? Of course he wanted to reduce his own responsibility in these crimes ... he was facing death row.

And, by the way, Bundy's crimes were committed decades before the web even existed.

Campaigns like the one against 'extreme' porn are nothing new. Cheap and readily available printing in the mid-nineteenth century led to the popularisation of stories and true crime tales among a mostly young male audience. Called 'penny dreadfuls', they were widely blamed for glorifying violence to working-class readers. Mary Whitehouse's campaign against 'video nasties' in the 1980s exploited a similar discomfort with new technology. The widely publicised campaign not only demonised something that was never shown to cause any particular crime, it also spread the distribution of such videos to a far larger audience than they would have otherwise enjoyed. In many ways, such public decency campaigns against new technological entertainments often have the exact opposite effect than was intended.

Opponents of the extreme porn law feared that it would target consumers of fetish porn, since the legislation makes no distinction between consenting and non-consenting participants. It also targeted animal porn, but made no distinction between live animals, cartoons of animals, or people dressed as animals (so-called 'furries').

Other critics of the law on violent porn were concerned that it was wide open to abuse by the police. There are technicalities of law that, instead of being enforced in the spirit in which they were written, are also commonly used against anyone who is investigated for unrelated reasons – think Al Capone and tax evasion. Given how much inappropriate material is viral in nature and can easily appear on your phone or in your email without you wanting to see it, this could criminalise a lot of ordinary people. Would it be possible for people to be prosecuted for material they never sought out?

The confusion doesn't end there. While films classified by the British Board of Film Classification are exempt from the legislation, stills from the same films are not. So the 2009 cinema release of *Antichrist* by Lars von Trier, which features a scene of a woman performing female genital mutilation on herself, would be fine. But a single frame of the scene taken from the film would be potentially illegal.

The Labour government answered critics of the extreme porn law by saying that it was meant to target only those whose porn habits were a serious concern. The spirit of the law was supposed to be to prevent murders similar to Jane Longhurst's. So, has the law worked? Has it prevented another terrible death like Jane's, or put away another disturbed criminal like Graham Coutts?

No. The prosecutions associated with the new law have not targeted potentially murderous obsessives. Rather, it has been used to bring additional charges in cases completely unrelated to sex crime. The way the law is written means anyone in possession of just one 'extreme' image could be charged, regardless of how the image came into their possession.

Perusing cases in which the law has been used shows such misuses have already happened. Take for instance Andrew Holland, who was prosecuted for a joke animation he was sent starring Tony the Tiger. Or Michael Nelson in Sunderland, who was arrested for unrelated offences when police found two short video clips that had been sent unsolicited to his phone. It turned out both of them have been in wide circulation on the internet for at least ten years. Extreme violence? Or common-or-garden tasteless humour? Juries never got to see the clips and decide, since that interpretation is strictly up to the judge.

In both the Holland and the Nelson cases, the law was used to bring charges despite the lack of any evidence that the men involved were thought to be sex predators. Not for the first time, a law is being used as a way of getting an arrest where there is not enough evidence to pursue the original investigation.

The evidence that porn does not cause violence is ample, but it's a message that has yet to penetrate the newsrooms of Britain. 'The cycle of addiction leads one way: towards ever harder material,' claims Edward Marriott in the *Guardian*. As evidence he makes reference to 'the now-infamous Carnegie Mellon study of porn on the internet,' which 'found that images of hardcore sex were in far less demand than more extreme material'.[96]

Unfortunately for Marriott, the study he mentions has been widely debunked. 'Marketing Pornography on the Information Superhighway' was a high-profile piece that looked at Usenet groups.[97] Its shocking results were widely publicised – until duped journalists for *Time* magazine and other media outlets were sheepishly forced to admit that it had all been made up. Academics whose names had been associated with the research were quick to distance themselves from it.[98] It's pretty surprising for someone to know about that article and not know about it being discredited so publically.

As once went 'penny dreadfuls' and 'video nasties', so now goes the common thinking about the effects of the internet. Placing blame at the door of technology ignores the fact that horrid sex crimes like the murder of Jane Longhurst are, and remain, thankfully rare. Cutting off the porn supply will not prevent another death – killers like Graham Coutts and Vincent Tabak existed long before the internet.

When law is written quickly, either in response to a perceived crisis or in order to bolster a government or further an agenda, there is always the risk that it will be used more for harm than good.

Take, for instance, the October 2011 announcement from Prime Minister David Cameron that he was meeting with internet service providers to discuss filtering content. The assumption is that an opt-in system would be an effective way to keep young people from looking at adult materials. Quite apart from the civil rights questions raised from keeping a database of the people who want to look at pornography online, there are a number of other issues.

Will it be an effective filter? Unlikely. The web alone is growing at such a vast rate that the only sensible way to filter material is by using programs to screen content rather than actual people. This can lead to unintended blocks. Famously, back in the early 1990s, some AOL users received warnings for discussing 'tits' in online forums. They were twitchers talking about birds, not sex fiends slavering over women.

Many wonder what such a ban would actually look like. Recently, I had a direct experience showing why these filters are bound to fail.

A friend on Twitter pointed out that a story about internet porn on the *Daily Mail* website in fact contained an image of someone looking at a computer monitor, and on that monitor was an actual pornographic image.[99] Knowing my phone's browser was supposed to automatically detect and block adult material, I decided to see if I could view the page in question. If the block was effective, then in theory, I shouldn't have been able to see the image or even open the page.

That's not exactly what happened. I could see it just fine, naked lady and all. It was another few hours before the *Mail* website altered the image to blur the porn, but still, you can imagine plenty of similar instances in which objectionable material would sail past the authorities.

Then, on a hunch, I decided to do some more phone browsing. I have a friend who is an SRE (sex and relationships education) specialist. His site, which contains no explicit images and very little rude talk, is designed specifically as a safe resource for teens and their parents. What do you know? Blocked on the phone's browser. And all I would have to do in order to unblock it is go to my phone company's nearest shop, present a copy of my passport to prove my age (which they already have from when I signed the contract with them), and pay for access to a site that is free on other browsers. Way to profit from a panic!

There must be loads of other people who would have similar problems … cancer researchers blocked from searching the word 'breast' – something that used to happen on NHS computers when I was in science. Rape victims unable to find online information about vital services. The capacity for such top-down measures to fail the users is almost unimaginably large.

But the 'ban the filth' juggernaut continues whether we actually need it or not. With confused ideas about cause and effect, and a mysterious Agenda Setter guiding politicians, what is the public to make of all of this?

People are often unaware of the origins of the scare tactics deployed by the media Evangelisers. And with the majority of the public in no position to critique the bogus statistics properly themselves, cargo cult science wins the day yet again.

Unfortunately, there is little to make headlines in statements such as 'we should consider the social and developmental concerns of a ten-year-old and a fifteen-year-old to be rather different' when discussing young people and internet use. Or 'people with different environments and different circumstances often interpret the same cues differently' when talking about whether porn ever really is a good enough defence against a murder charge. It's far too boring a bit of nuance for the media. And, sadly, it seems far too boring for the people advising the government, as well.

By looking at basic criteria to do with some of the scare stories and rigged statistics making the rounds, we can see that an agenda of legislating online access features in virtually every discussion. But that raises the grim possibility of the state deciding what is and is not appropriate. While they have a legitimate interest in protecting people, there is simply nothing in the assumption that tightening online materials reduces sex crimes or harm to children.

Certainly young people are living within a different time to the one their parents grew up in. There is easier access to sexualised (and often commercialised) messages. These are not just within the domains of 'internet porn' but often in the pages of our daily papers, celebrity sex scandal stories, music, advertising, and so on. It is important to talk about the information both young people and parents need, but deciding to begin this debate by recommending a top-down, censoring approach does not allow us to really explore what would help young people and where actual risks may originate.

As citizens, and as families, we should be asking harder questions when the debate comes up ... of who will decide where the line is, what their credentials are to make these decisions, and how we feel about that.

7

MYTH: Tens of thousands of women are trafficked into Britain as sex slaves.

I n the years after the Berlin Wall fell, Eastern European gangs set up operations to smuggle highly profitable items, like drugs, guns, cigarettes. And women. They usually transported young women from their hometowns in the Eastern Bloc south to Greece. Once successfully inside Greece, the women could be transported within the EU without being stopped at the borders.

As stories of sex trafficking in mainland Europe emerged, people became concerned about Eastern European women coming to Britain. Were they the usual economic migrants, working as call girls for ready cash? Or were they part of a more sinister trend, being controlled by gangs of thugs? It was hard to tell who was coming to the UK on their own for the money ... and who was being forced into working as a prostitute.

In the absence of any sensible figures, people assumed the worst in all cases. The conventional wisdom was that the women were being trafficked. Government agencies, police forces, and charities joined forces – and obtained funding – to deal with what they claimed was a widespread, insidious criminal trend. Numbers that were inflated, misreported, or in some cases completely made up and wrong started to circulate as if they were fact.

Now, no one supports kidnap or rape in any circumstances. Where forced sex trafficking occurs, and it does occur, it is a heinous crime against the women (and men) who are its victims.

At the same time, there are people who have manipulated the facts to suit various agendas. By presenting the issues as strictly black and white, they have laid claim to the moral high ground. In virtually everything written about trafficking, the victims are by and large women, by and large used for sex. But the majority of real trafficking cases are in fact not like this at all. Sound science must be our guide in choosing which problems to tackle and how to approach them.

No one would ever argue about whether or not forced sex work is right, or whether it occurs. It's very wrong, and it does happen. The point is that the closer we look at the truth about trafficking, the more we find not women and children being saved from terrible fates, but powerful Agenda Setters and misguided Constellation Makers claiming money and attention for themselves. They often focus solely on women and sex workers, and they often have an agenda against sex work and want to outlaw it even for consenting adults.

Meanwhile, Evangelisers step in, spreading fear and panic, yet rarely coming back to correct mistakes or admit to errors later. Open any newspaper or magazine, and the story is the same. 'Sex Slave in Suburbia', a May 2010 article in *Glamour* magazine, claimed there are half a million women trafficked in the EU for sex. Is the number even plausible? As far as figures go, it's absurdly high. And no source for the number is offered.

The article goes on to claim that punters are 'more likely' to visit a trafficked sex worker than a non-trafficked one, though police records and research do not back this up. Again, where exactly *Glamour* got this juicy titbit from is anyone's guess. Women's glossy magazines aren't the only ones who have been throwing improbably high figures around, and surely they must be getting their numbers from somewhere. So, where is all the misinformation coming from?

The problem starts with a deceptively simple question: how many trafficked sex workers are there in the UK? It's an easy question to ask, but almost impossible to answer. That hasn't stopped people who have claimed – wrongly – to know the answer from quoting unrealistic totals, though. How the desperate fate of a few unlucky women became one of the starkest examples of media hype and exaggeration is a very interesting tale.

In 2009, Labour MP Denis MacShane wrote a letter to the *Guardian* claiming 18,000 young women were trafficked into Britain 'as sex slaves'. Later he told Parliament that the number was in fact 25,000. The source for these numbers was reportedly a Home Office document.[100]

However, some doubted the figure was accurate. The then solicitor general, Vera Baird, challenged MacShane and his supposed source, the *Daily Mirror*. She claimed that the real number of women was closer to 4000.

But, as it turns out, even this was a major exaggeration. This is the story of how a speculative number tentatively suggested by researchers became a vastly inflated 'truth'. It involves media and government and misinformation – with each iteration of the story straying further and further from reality. And, ironically, potentially putting at risk the very lives they intend to save.

It's time to shed a little light on who is generating this expensive moral panic – and what they stand to gain from it.

Human trafficking is a challenging problem. Once brought into a country, trafficked people rarely turn up on the radar unless crime or death is involved. When nineteen Chinese cocklers drowned in Morecambe Bay in 2004, it highlighted the appalling conditions forced workers live in. Of the survivors, nine were registered as asylum seekers and five were completely unknown to immigration services.

The majority of trafficking cases in the UK are, like that of the Chinese cocklers, unrelated to sex work. Media coverage equates all trafficking with sex trafficking, but most trafficked people are brought in for domestic labour, agriculture, and food processing. They end up in jobs British nationals don't want, or are hired by employers who want to illegally pay under the minimum wage. Vietnamese and Chinese children have been found working on UK cannabis farms, for example. And while the majority of trafficked workers are women, men make up about a quarter of all cases. The needs of trafficked men are rarely, if ever, addressed in discussion and policy. Putting the focus on such a specific subset of trafficking cases diverts both public attention and much-needed resources away from other forced labour problems.[101]

So, why the panic about women being trafficked for sex? Chinese cocklers travelling up and down the country, crammed into transit vans and sleeping dozens to a room, are invisible to most of us. The well-worn cliché of a damaged woman whose purity is compromised, on the other hand, tugs at the heartstrings more keenly than the abuse of mere 'economic migrants'.

Why is it so important to get the numbers right? Several reasons. First, there is intense competition over government grants for groups that assist victims of trafficking. Until recently, a large amount of this money went to groups such as the Poppy Project, which only serves female victims. So, if trafficking affects men as well, and occurs in work environments such as Morecambe Bay, there would be reasonable justification to question whether giving so much money to groups with such a narrow focus is necessarily a good idea.

Another reason is that trafficking puts a lot of pressure on police forces to try to combat the problem. From the point of view of anyone hoping to show encouraging or improved numbers in this aspect of crime control, it is far easier to focus on and target the sex industry than it is to address a problem that actually is not well understood and is far more diverse than most people think. It's understandable that with only so many bobbies on the beat, police forces want to conserve their resources. It's not necessarily the right approach, or a good one, but given the cutbacks the police are experiencing, it's no mystery why they take it.

Finally, it's hard to generate publicity for a problem if it's mainly experienced by people no one cares about. People who are poor and from overseas are *personae non gratae* in Britain, especially if they're perceived to be the cause of British job losses. With the majority of trafficked people working in domestic and labour industries, they are beneath contempt in the eyes of many. No one is overly fussed about their welfare. But women and – especially – children? Potentially being used for sex? Suddenly, you have a demographic people can be made to care about. Suddenly, you have the makings of a moral frenzy.

FIRST THINGS FIRST:
Not all trafficking is sex trafficking of women.

Of national referrals made in the UK in 2009,
74% were female, 26% were male.*

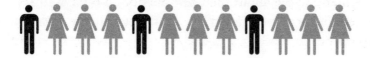

Sexual exploitation accounts for 43% (about four of every
ten) victims. Most are actually trafficked for manual and
domestic labour, for example in shops or on farms.†

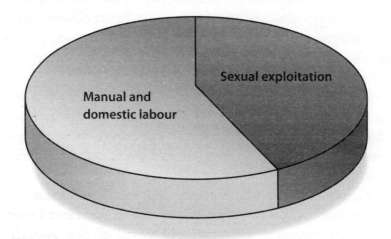

Sources:
* www.antislavery.org/includes/documents/cm_docs/2010/r/1_report_summary.pdf
† www.unglobalcompact.org/docs/issues_doc/labour/Forced_labour/HUMAN_TRAFFICKING_-_THE_FACTS_-_final.pdf

The popular opinion seems to be that someone trafficked for ordinary, non-sex work deserves whatever horror they get. But once sex is involved, the attitude changes dramatically.

Trafficking issues have a lot in common with the white slavery panics of the past. The term 'white slavery' was originally applied to both men and women, much like the term 'trafficking', in fact. But over time it became exclusively associated with sexual slavery of European women – again, in the way people now use 'trafficking' to mean only sexual trafficking of women and children. By narrowing the meaning from all people to a sympathetic few, it's possible not only to guide the discussion towards a specific agenda but also to whip up public outrage.

In the late nineteenth century, prostitution started to be seen as a pressing social problem, but also one that was strongly entrenched in society. While many wrote about the phenomenon, it took the campaigning of newspaperman William Thomas Stead in the 1880s to really engineer a public fervour. And as with many today, Stead did it not by addressing prostitution as a whole, but by focusing on an underground trade supposedly supplying young English girls to the upper classes. In fact, his writing and campaigns closely mirror the sort of stories peddled in the media today.

In 1885, Stead published a series of articles in the *Pall Mall Gazette*[102] called 'The Maiden Tribute of Modern Babylon'. Stead claimed there was a trade in virgins happening under the noses of the good people of London. He also recounted the sad story of a girl, Lily, sold by her mother for the purposes of prostitution.

'Almost every house of ill-fame in London is the centre of a network of snares and wiles and "plants", intended to bring in fresh girls,' Stead wrote. 'That is part of the regular trade.' Without presenting a single number or piece of evidence, he manages to claim that all brothels are doing it and it's happening everywhere.

The language of Stead's articles is over the top by today's standards. But it makes arguments that would not be out of place in any modern account of forced sex trafficking. 'London's lust annually uses up many thousands of women, who are literally killed and made away with,' Stead wrote. 'Living sacrifices slain in the service of vice.' He breathlessly describes 'the fatal chamber' in rich detail, with no observation too small or too unlikely to go unadorned with heavy prose. And the sex act itself is described in only the most florid terms, with a woman's virginity called 'that which a woman ought to value more than life'. It's practically pornographic in its focus on lurid detail.

Not only did Stead accuse rich Londoners of ignoring the problem, he claimed they were gleefully engaging in rape. He painted pictures of room after room of kidnapped women being flogged, much to their torturers' pleasure. 'To some men, the shriek of torture is the essence of their delight, and they would not silence by a single note the cry of agony over which they gloat.' As with so many modern campaigners, the assumption is that that men possess no feelings other than uncontrollable lust and inherent cruelty. Men with money, in particular.

The public uproar generated by the articles was enormous. The bookseller WH Smith initially refused to carry the papers because of the lascivious content. But the public demanded to know every last salacious detail. The stories were sold on the streets by the Salvation Army and used copies were re-sold at over ten times their cover price.

Stead revelled in his role, part Agenda Setter, part Constellation Maker, and without doubt a one-man Evangelising band. His campaign to end the Mills & Boon-esque drama he had whipped up culminated with hundreds of girls dressed in white marching on Parliament, encouraged by the *Gazette*, to demand a change in the age of consent from thirteen to sixteen. Because, for some reason, that was supposed to be all that was needed to stop the outrage. It seems charmingly naïve now to think something like changing age of consent laws could possibly have an effect if the dark and twisted underworld of London Stead painted in his paper week after week really had existed, but it was a hugely popular campaign, anyway.

As with so many supposedly black-and-white issues that people claim have simple answers, the truth of what Stead wrote about – and his involvement in the campaign – proved far murkier. While the trafficking stories he published were, on the face of it, successful, their very success backfired on him later.

Part of the problem with countering over-the-top claims like Denis MacShane's (and WT Stead's) is the lack of widely agreed statistics. Whatever number is presented, it's only an estimate. Illegal workers entering the country, whether forced or unforced labour, aren't exactly going to queue up at the border volunteering to be counted, are they? The question is, can we tell whether the numbers are an informed estimate or an uninformed guess?

Making estimates with limited information is called a 'Fermi problem'. Enrico Fermi, one of the physicists who worked on the Manhattan Project, was reputedly able to make accurate guesses at numbers others considered unknowable. The classic example was his estimate of how many piano tuners there are in Chicago. He was able to come up with an answer – 150 – that if not exact, was within a reasonable error margin.

Here's an example of a Fermi problem in action. I was at a pub quiz one week, and our team was tied for the lead. The tiebreaker was the question 'How many performances did Yul Brynner have as the King of Siam in *The King and I* on Broadway?' As the only former drama geek in our team, it came down to me. I calculated that Brynner probably did eight performances a week (once a day and twice on Sundays, as the saying goes). It's a full-time job, so minus a two-week holiday, Brynner was probably performing fifty weeks a year. I wasn't sure how many years the show ran for but knew he had been in at least one revival of the popular musical, so let's say ten years of being the king in total. That makes an estimate of:

$$8 \text{ shows a week} \times 50 \text{ weeks a year} \times 10 \text{ years} = 4000 \text{ shows}$$

Sounds pretty high, right? The other team probably thought so too, because they guessed 300. We won the tiebreak (and the quiz) because, as it turned out, the real answer is 4525. Picking a number out of thin air, as the other team did, is fraught with error. It's hard to make good guesses with no information. Apply some basic knowledge and your accuracy goes up rapidly.

Fermi problems are great for pub quizzes, but common-or-garden wild guesses are not always the stuff on which good research is built. At the very least, estimating a number should fulfil two major criteria:

1. **The assumptions must have some foundation in reality.** In the Yul Brynner example, eight Broadway performances a week is reasonable; eighty wouldn't be.

2. **The method of calculation needs to be explained.** I don't think the other person on my team would have supported 4000 as an answer if they hadn't seen my reasoning.

In forced sex trafficking estimates, most numbers have gone the other way: they've overcounted, rather than undercounted. The numbers of supposed sex slaves quoted by MacShane are so unrealistic that, if true, they would account for the vast majority of prostitution in Britain. Regardless of how you feel about sex work, there are self-evidently many non-immigrants in it. For instance, it is well known that the majority of street-based prostitutes in the UK are British, and almost all the rest are EU nationals. So his numbers are immediately suspect.

There are some decent estimates of the extent of sex work in the UK. As part of the European Network for HIV/STD Prevention in Prostitution (EUROPAP), Hilary Kinnell contacted projects providing services for sex workers. She had seventeen responses. The average number of prostitutes per project was 665. She then multiplied that figure by 120, the total number of projects on her mailing list, to get an estimate of 79,800. This total includes women, men, and transgender women and men.[103]

Hilary Kinnell is the first to point out the problems with her method: the centres responding might be larger than most, some sex workers might use more than one centre. She finds it strange that the number – ten years old, a huge estimate, and taken out of context – is still quoted. 'The figure was picked up by all kinds of people and quoted with great confidence but I was never myself at all confident about it. I felt it could be higher, but it also could have been lower.'

Meanwhile, data from the UK Network of Sex Work Projects (UKNSWP) records an estimate of 17,081 sex workers in some kind of contact with centres. Of these, 4178 – about 24 per cent – work on the street. A larger total for all sex workers was 48,393. More recent, and rather lower, than the 1999 estimate.[104] So, if the hype was real, that would mean anywhere from one in twelve to one in two sex workers was the victim of trafficking. However, a close examination of where those estimates came from shows this can't be true.

It all started with a study by Liz Kelly and Linda Regan of the University of North London. They attempted to estimate the number of women brought into the UK for sex in 1998 by surveying reports filed with police forces. The number they came up with was seventy-one.

Now, a note about that number: it included not only women who were trafficked against their will, but also women who was willingly arrived – perhaps illegally – to the UK for sex work. In other words, Kelly and Regan's total included both willing and unwilling sex migrants.

Part of the problem is how different groups define 'trafficked'. To many, the assumption was that if someone was not British and was working in the sex trade, she must be trafficked. That's quite a leap in logic! Hold on a sec – I was born abroad. And I worked in the sex trade. Does that mean they count me as 'trafficked'?

And the Kelly and Regan paper is not the only place such assumptions crop up. The Poppy Project reported in 2004 that 80 per cent of prostitutes in London flats were foreign-born. But there is no evidence that those women were trafficked or that this high proportion of foreign sex workers to natives is true of the entire UK. (In fact, evidence puts the UK-wide percentage of foreign-born sex workers closer to 37 per cent.)

If that still sounds high, keep in mind that 'foreign-born' also includes citizens of other EU countries, who have the automatic right to live and work in the UK. Not that these are always reported accurately. Eaves, the organisation that includes the Poppy Project, did an interesting nip-and-tuck on reporting the origins of women working in the sex trade in London. In their 2004 report *Sex in the City*, they claimed 25 per cent of women working in London were from Eastern Europe. But look closer – they have classified Italy and Greece as 'Eastern European' countries.[105]

Why? Well, the reason given is 'because these ethnicities are often used to code women from the Balkan region, advised by pimps and traffickers to lie about their ethnicity to avoid immigration issues.' Hey, my dad is Italian ... if I said this to a researcher, would they assume I'm lying, and am really Eastern European?

So, overall, when people talk about 'trafficked' women, what the number they quote more likely represents is 'foreign-born women who might have come here for other reasons, and who are probably in sex work by choice'. Rarely, if ever, is the definition of trafficking explained in the media. This violates the second principle of the realistic estimate: show your work clearly. It's the kind of sloppy calculation that throws all subsequent conclusions into question. It's bad Fermi.

So, if some people who come here voluntarily can be called 'trafficked', then what is 'trafficking', exactly? The *Palermo Protocol to Prevent, Suppress and Punish Trafficking in Persons Especially Women and Children*, part of the 2000 UN Convention against Transnational Organized Crime, defines 'trafficking' as:

> ... the threat or use of force or other forms of coercion, of abduction, of fraud, of deception, of the abuse of power or of a position of vulnerability or of the giving or receiving of payments or benefits to achieve the consent of a person having control over another person, for the purpose of exploitation.

In other words, illegal migration for purposes of economic advantage, if undertaken willingly and fully informed, is *not* trafficking.[106]

Nevertheless, because we don't know how many of those women were willing and how many were unwilling, let's assume the worst for the purpose of this Fermi problem. Let's assume every single one of those seventy-one women was brought to the UK (rather than emigrated) unwillingly. Kelly and Regan then grapple with underreporting. Without any hard information to go with, they guessed an equal number might have been missed by the police and doubled the seventy-one – so, a total of 142 women. That's the lower boundary of their estimate.

For the upper boundary, they guessed that trafficking might be undetected by a factor of as much as *twenty times*. So, the upper boundary of the estimate was 1420. The absolute maximum ... which, they emphasised, was speculative.

To summarise: the estimate for the absolute very highest number of trafficked women in this country for the year of 1998 was 1420. So, what do we know? That sex trafficking is possibly underreported, and no one knows the numbers, really. Still, even if the number is as small as the original number of seventy-one women per year, that is a clear breach of human rights – and an area

HOW THE NUMBERS GREW:
From 71 trafficked women to 25,000+.

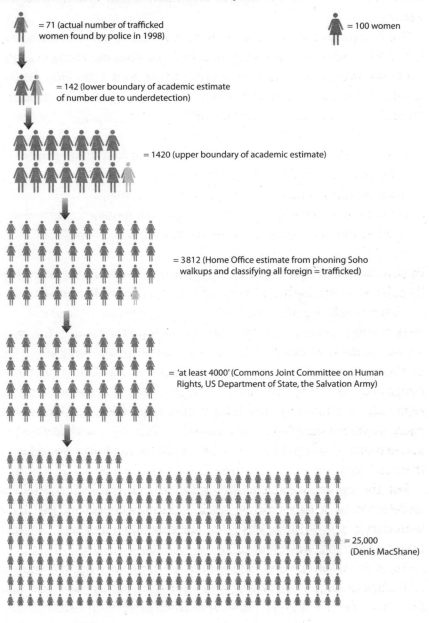

= 71 (actual number of trafficked women found by police in 1998)

= 100 women

= 142 (lower boundary of academic estimate of number due to underdetection)

= 1420 (upper boundary of academic estimate)

= 3812 (Home Office estimate from phoning Soho walkups and classifying all foreign = trafficked)

= 'at least 4000' (Commons Joint Committee on Human Rights, US Department of State, the Salvation Army)

= 25,000 (Denis MacShane)

about which the government should be concerned.

But that *highest possible* estimate of 1420 is considerably smaller – only about a third – of the number Vera Baird used. It is smaller than the claims made by MacShane by a factor of seventeen. How did that happen?

The journey from less than 1500 to 25,000 is an interesting one. At first, the original paper was cited with only a small error in reporting the results. Then the Salvation Army and Churches Alert to Sex Trafficking Across Europe (Chaste) reported not Regan and Kelly's range of values, but the estimated maximum value as if it were the number of *actual reports*. They updated the year as well – 'An estimated 1420 women were trafficked into the UK in 2000 for the purposes of constrained prostitution.'

Then, in 2003, the Home Office took inaccurate estimates a step further. Assuming *all* foreign-born women in Soho walkups to be trafficked, plus 75 per cent of foreign sex workers throughout the UK, plus 10 per cent of foreign call girls gave the total of 3812 women in forced sex work in Britain. Yes, this included even EU citizens who can travel and work here freely.

That number, rounded up to 4000 for no reason, is widely quoted without acknowledging that it is an inflation of someone else's highest possible number. And that is where Vera Baird's figure came from.

In 2006, the Commons Joint Committee on Human Rights heard this number entered into the Hansard as if it were a fact. Evangelisers with an anti-sex agenda now had the handy 'government figures showing' 4000 women being trafficked without the hassle of having to question whether that was actually true. Julie Bindel also claimed, '[S]tudies have found that at least 70 per cent of women working in UK brothels are trafficked from places such as Africa, Asia and Eastern Europe,' but in fact this had to be retracted later by the newspaper as no such study exists.[107]

The number 4000 also appeared in a US Department of State document on worldwide trafficking (although interestingly as a number representing all trafficking, not just sex trafficking).[108] The Christian charity Care picked up on it as well, and the Salvation Army replied by asserting the number was now *at least* 4000.

From there to 25,000 is actually only a matter of multiplying it by six and a bit, which was no doubt justified with some accusations of undercounting … in spite of the fact that the estimate used as the origin for all of these dodgy calculations was *itself* already an over-count. From what can be pieced together, it appears various groups and individuals have been happy to inflate the numbers along the way without ever questioning methods or sources.

When challenged to justify his number of 25,000 per year on *Newsnight*, Denis MacShane had no firm sources to hand.[109] He said he read it in the *Daily Mirror* and that it came from the Home Office, but the relevant article does not contain that claim.[110] MacShane was then forced to admit he did not know the origin of the numbers he was using.

Nick Davies, who reported on the phenomenon, commented, '… The cycle has been driven by political opportunists and interest groups in pursuit of an agenda … an unlikely union of evangelical Christians with feminist campaigners, who pursued the trafficking tale to secure their greater goal, not of regime change, but of legal change to abolish all prostitution.'[111]

Grahame Maxwell, chief constable for North Yorkshire, put the hype about sex-specific trafficking into perspective. 'There are more people trafficked for labour exploitation than there are for sexual exploitation. We need to redress the balance here. People just seem to grab figures from the air.'[112]

And what of the Eastern European women, whose sudden influx into the sex trade in Western Europe sparked recent concern about trafficking?

Only a few years ago, traffickers would send scouts into small towns to lure girls with promises of work abroad and force some of them into prostitution. But things have rapidly changed with the opening of Eastern European ports to the West … not to mention the rapid changes in the economy.

Today, few Eastern European prostitutes need to be tricked to enter the sex industry. Ports like Odessa, in southern Ukraine, have wit-nessed an above-ground boom in sex services. 'An experienced girl gets off the plane covered in gold, diamonds and furs, and goes back to her home village,' says psychologist Svetlana Chernolutskaya in an interview with *Time* magazine. 'She finds the girls who are in a tough spot and tells them how much money they can make turning tricks in a foreign country.'[113]

Leaked US diplomatic cables confirm that would-be rescuers hoping for glory in Armenia would be disappointed by the reality. 'We went to Vanadzor expecting to hear stories of illicit smuggling across borders and of girls lured into prostitution under false pretenses. What we heard was significantly more pedestrian ... And while the prostitutes and the NGO employees we met said sometimes women are abused in the brothels, or aren't paid in full, they said the greater part of women generally understand what they are getting themselves into, and may already have worked as prostitutes for years.'[114]

'Reporters always come here demanding to see the victims,' says Olga Kostyuk, deputy head of a charity providing help for Odessa's sex workers, in the same piece. 'They want to see the men, the pimps, the manipulators behind all of this. But things are not so simple now.'

Indeed, television crews looking for simple answers can quickly find themselves perpetrating a hoax. In 2008, an ITV programme related the tale of a fourteen-year-old girl sold for sex at a petrol station in Romania. The problem was, it wasn't true. The woman was actually twenty-five years old. And a career sex worker.

In the report, broadcast worldwide on CNN, an ITV journalist claimed Monica Ghinga's identification papers proved she was fourteen years old. The journalist met with alleged traffickers, saying he would pay €800 for her and take the girl to London. Romanian police discovered the truth when they investigated the television claims, to see if forced child trafficking was really involved.

Ghinga later admitted that she lied about her age to a foreign television crew, and agreed to have sex with them for one night.[115] A claim that, if true, throws into question just who is taking advantage of whom in the trafficking panic.

WT Stead's nineteenth-century claims about sex slavery were successful for several reasons. Rather than focus on the trade of girls outside of Britain, Stead's exposé took place right under the noses of his readers – right in the heart of London. The same is true of anti-trafficking proponents today. There is far more concern about sex slavery in the EU than in the rest of the world, even though it has been shown to be far more prevalent elsewhere.

Instead of being concerned with the daughters of the unsympathetic poor, Stead's victims were from the new middle class. There is now, as then, something more sympathetic about the thought of attractive, innocent girls being exploited. Weirdly enough, if you do an image search of anti-trafficking campaign posters and billboards, one trend is immediately apparent: that most of them depict naked, bound women, usually very good-looking, in some form or other.

Now, don't get me wrong ... I like a little bondage as much as the next person. But really? How is anyone meant to take the message to stop exploiting women seriously, when the image itself is exploitation? I'm not sure if they're trying to educate their intended audience, or titillate them. Looks like the latter to me.

Stead portrayed aristocrats as being secret consumers of prostitution, with access to virgins for the best connected and most well heeled. Again, modern campaigners like to claim that access to trafficked women is in brothels or by invitation only (that's why no one can prove it exists.)

Crucially, Stead declared that a change in the age of consent was not only necessary, but sufficient to end the horror. This is a key element of his campaign's success. He worked as an Agenda Setter, Constellation Maker, and Evangeliser all rolled into one. He not only described a problem, but also manufactured the evidence and proposed a solution to eradicate it. People like to believe things can be easily solved. Today, the popular impression is that criminalising prostitution is all that is needed to end trafficking.

The current debate has followed many similar lines to previous panics: keep the focus at home, instead of overseas. Portray the victims as unknowing innocents, instead of unsympathetic addicts or poor. And if no one is able to detect the problem? Easy. That's because the bad guys are evil plutocrats who have the resources to keep their unsavoury habits well hidden. The solution? Very simple: total crackdown.

In 2007, police forces across the country started a wide-scale investigation into sex trafficking. Called Pentameter Two, it was hailed by Jacqui Smith as 'a great success'. Claims were made that it exposed nationwide crime networks and was directly responsible for rescuing vulnerable women. With the co-operation of all fifty-five police forces in England, Wales, Scotland, and Northern Ireland, the Border Agency and the Crown Prosecution Service, you would expect the result to be nothing short of comprehensive.

What Smith and others failed to mention was that this all-encompassing operation, using every method at police disposal, including brothel raids, undercover operations, and co-ordinated information, was not successful. As Nick Davies detailed in a series of articles for the *Guardian*, Pentameter Two resulted in five convictions of men accused of importing women and forcing them to work as prostitutes. Five convictions across the entire country.

A total of 406 arrests were made during Pentameter Two; 153 of those people were released without charge. Most of the rest were charged with immigration breaches and unrelated offences. Twenty-two were prosecuted for trafficking; seven of those were acquitted. Ten of the remaining lot turned out not to have coerced the women they brought into the country. This left five actual traffickers.[116] And, it was later revealed, none of those was detected specifically by actions in the Pentameter Two effort, but due to other investigations.

In terms of finding and stopping traffickers, Pentameter Two failed to be responsible for even one trafficking conviction. Still, the operation had another aspect: not only finding the people involved in trafficking, but also rescuing the women themselves.

So, how well did it do on that count? During operations Pentameter Two in 2008 and its predecessor Pentameter One in 2006, over 1300 locations were raided. A total of 255 women were 'rescued'. That suggests that the proportion of forced women in sex work is far lower than the 80 per cent claimed by Fiona Mactaggart MP. (Who, it turns out, was using as her source of information a survey of street-based sex workers. In San Francisco. From 1982.[117])

Were they trafficked? As ever, the question is hard to answer, especially since by late 2009, police had lost track of most of them.[118] Of the 255 women, 16 were deported, 36 of them returned home, and 37 accepted victim support services. The whereabouts of the rest – 166 women – are unknown.

It seems that the 255 women, rather than being the victims of involuntary trafficking, were voluntary migrants. Dr Belinda Brooks-Gordon at Birkbeck College specialises in sexuality and the law, and she commented on the phenomenon. 'We do know a lot of women in the former Russian states who are working in sex industry and who are desperate to come here. They want to earn more money here – they are migrant workers like any other workers.'

In Northern Ireland, with similar efforts, the numbers again turn out to be far smaller than expected. With 25 cases of human trafficking in 2009/2010, 17 of which involved sexual exploitation – the number of trafficking victims is less than 1 per 100,000 people.[119] And again, the terminology is vague – is being exploited for sex the same thing as being forced into sex? After all, one could argue the employees of fast-food restaurants are exploited ... but no one would say they are forced. From the reported figures it's tough to say if even this basic distinction was made.

Still, even if only a small number of sex traffickers are operating in this country, that should be cause for worry, and who could disagree? In theory, yes. If police funding and time were unlimited, every crime should be investigated to the utmost.

But Pentameter Two was not a case of unlimited money, or of people, or of time. Police forces were made to take part but no additional money and staff were provided. Funding is allocated under the Reflex project, which receives £20 million a year, but with no specific provision for Pentameter Two.[120] In other words, police forces were required to conduct undercover investigations and raids – in addition to whatever trafficking-detection activities they already carried out – without any extra support. In a practical sense, this is a diversion of resources that resulted in not one fresh conviction.

In the opinion of Professor Julia O'Connell Davidson, lawmakers should be angry about the failure of Pentameter. Let's go back to Denis MacShane's huge estimate of 25,000 trafficked sex slaves from the *Daily Mirror*. That story claimed women were forced to have sex with thirty men a day. If true, that means 750,000 men exploit sex slaves every day. That's huge.

'How is it that three-quarters of a million men can find a sex slave every day but when highly trained police officers run a special nation-wide operation lasting months they can only find at best a couple of hundred women that they think might be victims of trafficking?' asked O'Connell Davidson on Radio 4.[121] At the very least it represents money wasted on either mass incompetence or mass misunderstanding of the problem.

Pentameter One and Two aren't the only wastes of police time and money in this moral panic. Other projects have resulted in similarly inflated projections, also with underwhelming results.

Project Acumen, set up by the Association of Chief Police Officers (ACPO), released its findings in 2010. Titled *Setting the Record*, the report focuses on sex trafficking and where the people come from, as well as their circumstances.[122]

Based on this, the *Telegraph* claimed 12,000 'confirmed' trafficked women were in the UK.[123] It goes on: 'In a typical example, a woman smuggled into the UK does not know that she is going to be used as a prostitute, but is forced into selling her body to pay off a £30,000 "debt-bond".'

Does the report actually say this? It doesn't. And where does 12,000 come from? It's not clear.

Project Acumen's report didn't locate 12,000 women, much less interview anything like that many. It is actually based on interviews with 210 foreign and 44 British sex workers located at 142 premises in England and Wales. Of the 210 migrants, none was kidnapped or held hostage. Only one was the victim of violence.

Most of the migrants – 202 of the 210 – knew at the time of recruitment that they would be working as prostitutes in the UK. Of the other eight, it is unclear whether they were misled about location rather than the work. Two dozen were labelled trafficked – nineteen Asians and five Eastern Europeans. The criteria, however, were not determined by the UN's Palermo Protocol, but by a complex set of 'dimensions', that again, do not seem to distinguish willing (if perhaps illegal) migration from unwilling trafficking.

Only a small percentage of the women were considered 'debt-bonded' – owing money to those who had brought them to the UK. These debts could be because of transport costs, or monies owed by their families. Hardly a 'typical' example, as the paper claimed.

The number 12,000 pops up in the report – an estimate of about 4000 trafficked sex slaves pulled out of thin air, with 8000 more from 'vulnerable' populations. Again, no reliable sources for these numbers exist. Interestingly the paper qualifies its statements with 'Most are likely to fall short of the trafficking threshold.' Or, in other words, there is no way to prove their claims either way. Of the made-up number, it continues:

> Approximately 3,700 of them are from Asia; there may be significant cultural factors which prevent them from exiting prostitution or seeking help, but they tend to have day-to-day control over their activities and do not consider themselves to be debt-bonded. A further estimated 4,100 are from Eastern Europe; although many are legally entitled to live and work in the UK, they tend to speak little English and because they live and work in areas they are unfamiliar with they are overly reliant on their controllers. Most made a conscious decision to become involved in prostitution, albeit with limited alternatives, and the financial rewards on offer are considered to be a significant pull factor for these individuals.

Plenty of speculation, and very little sense. And, no doubt, considerable spending on a project that many taxpayers may find wasteful. After all, this report is the culmination of two years' study, and found very few women, a tiny fraction of whom met the threshold circumstances of forced sex trafficking. Pentameter Two found barely any more potentially trafficked women in the entire country … and no actual sex slaves. The whole outcome has the whiff of what Dr Belinda Brooks-Gordon, a reader in psychology and social policy at Birkbeck, has called 'Carry-On Criminology'.

Figures from the UK Human Trafficking Centre confirm that the number of trafficked women is far smaller than is widely reported. In the 12-month period from April 2009 to March 2010, 709 referrals were made to the centre, with the majority detected by border control rather than police. Of the 709 in that year, just 319 were referred as suspected cases of sex trafficking. Only about half the cases had been processed by the time of the report, but of those, 68 per cent were dismissed as not trafficking.[124]

Even before the failure of Pentameter Two it could have been predicted that the projected numbers were not only inflated, but also conceptually unfeasible. This is partly to do with the difficulty of getting past British borders – despite what the immigration panickers think, it's still harder to get into the UK than anywhere else in the EU. But also there is a near total absence of sex tourism in this country.

Sex tourism in countries with land borders is straightforward, and its existence in mainland Europe well documented over the last couple of decades. Consider Eastern Europe, within easy reach of Poland, Germany, the Czech Republic, and other EU countries. If you want to get to a thriving area of sex workers, it's only a short flight or drive away. Sex tourism is also popular in areas where British pounds go a bit further than they do at home: places like Cuba and Thailand.

Sex tourism to the UK, however, is rather implausible. In an age of cheap international flights from Britain to virtually anywhere, and ample numbers of women at home who go into the work willingly, it makes no financial sense for traffickers to bring women here for sex when they could operate more easily, and with a more ready supply of customers, in mainland Europe or the developing world.

This logic is supported by the results of investigation. After all, Pentameter Two, to date the most wide-ranging investigation of sex trafficking in the UK, failed to result in enough evidence to suggest that anything remotely resembling a crisis is happening here. That poster girl for the Trafficking Panic, the wide-eyed teenage girl kidnapped into a life of ill repute, is not representative. She is nearly an urban myth.

Short-term failure has never stopped Agenda Setters. When the disappointing outcome was revealed, some people claimed Pentameter Two was not a failure at all. 'Pentameter Two has been a great success,' claimed Nick Kinsella, head of the UK Human Trafficking Centre. 'Now the results need to be analysed in depth, to see what we have actually found.' Wait, what was that? It's been a great success, only no one knows what the numbers say yet?

'In Scotland, to the best of my knowledge, we don't have a conviction for human trafficking,' said Police Constable Gordon Meldrum. Meldrum had previously claimed research 'proved' the existence of 10 human trafficking groups north of the border, and 367 organised crime groups with over 4000 members. 'We had one case which was brought to court previously but was abandoned. My understanding is it was abandoned due to a lack of evidence, essentially.'[125] Strange how the evidence seemed to disappear precisely when someone was charged with putting cases together.

Others invoked fiction to explain shortfalls. 'The Wire,' wrote Catherine Bennett in the *Observer*, 'showed just how tricky it can be when, with the best of intentions, the authorities attempt to organise human squalor.'[126] *The Wire* was a television series about criminals and police in Baltimore, Maryland. It was critically lauded for showing how investigations can fail because of lack of political motivation. One series even had a storyline about trafficked women who suffocated while being smuggled in a shipping container.

And yet, *The Wire*, for all its gritty semblance of reality, is not a documentary and no reflection of the situation in Britain. Pentameter 2 received explicit government support, was co-ordinated across police areas, and diverted large amounts of resources. Assuming that the kind of bureaucratic red tape and farcical errors encountered in a US-based drama are an insight into police work in Britain is an argument that is at best lazy and at worst laughable.

Since we're talking about America, let's compare trafficking panics here with similar stings in the US – and the reality there.

The US has a much higher population than the UK, and vast unguarded land borders with other countries, which have been customarily exploited for drug running and illegal migration.

Portland is a city in the Northwestern US state of Oregon. It's the state's largest, lying about 150 miles south of Seattle, Washington along the same highway. The quality of living is high: Portland is frequently named one of the US's best cities to live in for its easy accessibility, robust economy, and access to nature.

In 2010 and 2011, the city became an unexpected target of reports on sex trafficking. Respected newsreader Dan Rather dubbed the city

'Pornland'. Others called it the 'epicentre for child prostitution' and a 'hotbed of sex trafficking'. Actors such as Daryl Hannah and politicians descended for the Northwest Conference Against Trafficking to discuss what should be done to get this pervasive problem under control.

In November 2010, Portland's mayor, Sam Adams, declared to the press that his city had become 'stained' as a centre of sex trafficking. Portland police, he claimed, report an average of two cases of child sex trafficking every week.

The problem with the number? It isn't true.

According to Sergeant Mike Geiger of the Portland Sex Crimes Unit, police don't track such statistics. 'I am not sure where that is coming from,' he said. 'That's an unreliable number.'[127] So how did Portland become the focus of a moral panic?

In February 2009, an FBI investigation in Portland found seven prostitutes under the age of eighteen. This caught the media's attention in a big way, and they claimed strip clubs and permissive attitudes led middle-class girls to be tricked into prostitution. With no indication of how many of the seven girls were actually trafficked, it was naturally assumed they all must have been.

Another FBI sting in October 2009 found four girls under eighteen. Politicians scrambled to do something. (A similar operation found sixteen underage girls in Seattle, but no one seemed as concerned about Seattle as they were about friendly, trendy, middle-class Portland.)

A frequently cited claim is that 300,000 youths in the US, Canada, and Mexico are at risk of sexual exploitation.[128] The US Department of Justice cites this statistic, as do UNICEF, CNN, and the National Center for Missing and Exploited Children. However, over time, Evangelisers have begun to cite the number 300,000 as an actual count of trafficked US-only children.

There are two problems. First, being at risk of exploitation does not mean that all, or even many, of those young people will be sexually exploited. Of those who are, there no reason to think all, or even most, will be trafficked for paid sex. For instance the report itself confirms that 'Nearly all of it [sexual exploitation] occurs in the privacy of the child's own home (84%) ... 96% of all confirmed child sexual abuse cases are perpetrated by persons known either to the child or to the child's family.' Instances of abuse are rarely caused by strangers snatching children from their beds in the night, and yet that seems to be the only thing people are concerned about.

What do the authors consider a risk? Well, the tally includes such categories as children of migrants, for instance – in spite of the questionable assumption that immigration is a risk factor for child sexual abuse.

The study took data counting the number of runaways under eighteen. The authors then came up with a percentage they believed to be at risk of sexual exploitation based on interviews with fewer than 300 teens. Unsurprisingly, other statistics from the same report, such as 'Only about 10% of the [confirmed sexually exploited] children we encountered are trafficked internationally' are not often mentioned. In any case, extrapolating from such a small group to cover all young people over an entire continent is statistically problematic and not a good basis for a nationwide estimate.

The other problem is that in spite of extensive efforts against trafficking, the number of confirmed sex trafficking incidents in the US does not even come close to the overinflated figures. Just as in the UK.

The US Bureau of Justice reports that between 1 January 2007 and 30 September 2008 task forces reported investigating 1229 alleged incidents of human trafficking.[129] Sex trafficking accounted for 1018 (83 per cent) of the alleged incidents. Of these, 391 (38 per cent) involved allegations of child sex trafficking.

Less than 10 per cent of the reported incidents turned out to be human trafficking. Allegations of forced adult prostitution accounted for 63 per cent of the rejected investigations that were ultimately found not to involve human trafficking elements.

Over 21 months, in a country with 5 times the population of Britain and far easier ports of entry, only 120 cases of human trafficking were confirmed. That's less than six per month for the entire country. If we scale the results by population, this makes confirmed trafficking in Britain and the US very similar to each other. It also indicates trafficking is very rare in both countries.

Most of the US cases did not involve foreigners: 63 per cent of those 'rescued' in confirmed trafficking cases were US citizens.[130] Of that

120, it is unclear how many were women, if any were underage, and – crucially – how much of the trafficking was for the purposes of sex. Remember, the number of people trafficked for labour far outnumber the number trafficked for sex.

The results suggest two things: the laws regarding trafficking and border control are tough enough to ensure it is easier for such criminals to stay outside US and UK borders, and the rewards for this business are sufficiently low that there is not enough motivation for gangs to subvert those laws.

Now, it is possible, even likely, that there are more people being trafficked than are being found by the raids. There are two reasons why this might happen. One is a focus on sex work as the exclusive result of forced labour. The second is the tendency for police raids to treat people as criminals first, and potential victims second.

Consider anti-trafficking efforts in the US, where sex work is illegal. As with the UK, most police raids focus on brothels and massage parlours – not factories or farms, the type of sites where most trafficking violations occur. But the raids are not even effective at identifying trafficked women within the trade. The Sex Workers Project, a US charity, interviewed women who *had* been trafficked.[131] They report that 60 per cent of those women had been arrested in raids, some as many as ten times. None had been identified as trafficked at the time of their arrest. Only one was asked whether she was coerced into sex. Even in raids looking for victims, women in the sex industry are treated as criminals first.

These raids and arrests do not address the needs of people who may actually be trafficked, but rather the presuppositions of those who claim to be helping. There has been little focus on identifying what potential victims of crime would actually find helpful and effective. A human-rights-based approach to trafficking would prioritise the needs of potential victims over criminal justice.

With Agenda Setters and Evangelisers at the helm of a crusade, the government can easily be convinced to change laws. Politicians' understanding of the evidence is limited, especially if they see a shocking statistic in a newspaper, if it sounds plausible, and it fits with their world view. It is easier to follow a high-profile campaigner than to question the lack of evidence. They might even be tempted to exaggerate numbers themselves in order to further the cause.

In the case of Victorian newspaperman WT Stead, success in his campaign to change the age of consent resulted in near ruin. Rival journalists discovered that his story of Lily's sale was really a story about Stead himself buying a girl named Eliza. Stead did this because he could find no other evidence for the scenarios he wrote about so convincingly. The law he had promoted to change the age of consent was then used to prosecute him. It emerged that he had lied to the girl's mother, saying Eliza would become a servant to a rich family. His stories had claimed that the mother was complicit in selling her child into sex slavery.

What Stead and other opponents of prostitution aim to do is combine the many issues around migration and crime into a single focus. Trafficking has ceased to refer, in the popular imagination, to anything but young women and sex. Victorian reformers recast the image of all prostitutes as victims of forces beyond their control; the same happens now.

Slowly some people have started to pick up on the real numbers, but is anyone in power listening? 'Everybody says that there are a tremendous number of trafficked women in Britain, but we have no idea of the figures,' said former MP Anthony Steen. 'The human trafficking centre in Sheffield … spends nearly £2 million a year, but we ain't got the numbers. We do not know how many people are involved. It is pure guesswork and sensationalism when people talk about 4000 to 6000. The figure is probably in the hundreds, not the thousands.'[132] Certainly the outcomes of Pentameter Two and Project Acumen support his analysis.

In the US as well, huge amounts of effort and money are being spent to attack a problem that may not exist. In Portland, with fewer than twenty under-eighteen prostitutes in a year and no idea how many (if any) were trafficked, local government used the publicity to net $500,000 in federal grants to fight commercial sexual exploitation, including a computer system to track cases.

Politicians claimed the area was 'particularly attractive to traffickers', leading to a 'particularly high prevalence of sexual exploitation of children'. In spite of assurances from the FBI that Portland's problem is no greater than other cities', and no evidence that the teen-agers were in sex work by force. Meanwhile, commissioners allocated $7 million to local governments to fight the 'problem' and $900,000 for a Portland shelter. On the basis of eleven girls – none of whom were confirmed as trafficked – about $8 million will be allocated to fight the 'epidemic'.

Unfortunately, the disproportionate waste of time and money has not dissuaded the perpetrators of moral panic. Operation Monaco, a crackdown on sexual services advertised in phone boxes, was launched in London in March 2009. The raids resulted in, as the *News of the World* tittered, an 'array of sex toys (in addition to the array of bankers): nipple clamps, handcuffs and patent leather stiletto boots, as well as a wardrobe full of rubber uniforms – including nurse outfits.'[133] It also resulted in only one charge of controlling a prostitute for gain, and photos of sex workers who were never charged with any crime splashed across the Sunday tabloids.[134] Whether the failure of these operations and the inaccuracy of the trafficking estimates will have any effect on those who profit from them remains to be seen.

Even Antislavery International has gone so far as to say, 'Evidence shows that current measures have not improved the rate of trafficking convictions in the UK, and in some cases they actively undermine prosecutions.'[135]

Any person – especially a young person – trafficked for any reason is a cause for concern. But overstating the problem can actually harm victims rather than help them. It also does a disservice to the victims of other types of trafficking to concentrate only on sex. There are real traffickers operating in the EU, probably secure in the knowledge that the main focus is not on them.

The way these investigations are carried out is also unlikely to win any allies from within the sex industry. Meenu Seshu, founder of SANGRAM, a peer education organisation for sex workers in India, summarises the situation: 'The community is never, ever going to respond to anybody who is bringing in the police to rescue them, because they do not view that as a "rescue". They view that as another oppressive thing that's done to them.'[136]

In other countries, trafficking crackdowns have not only failed, they have put non-trafficked sex workers at risk.

In Cambodia, the government began targeting the sex industry with its 2008 Law on Suppression of Human Trafficking and Sexual Exploitation. A survey last year found that less than 1 per cent of sex workers in Cambodia were sold into prostitution.[137] The trafficking panic has nonetheless overshadowed the health and human rights of the other 99 per cent of Cambodian sex workers – with potentially deadly results.

The unintended consequences are massive. Organisations battling the high rate of HIV in Cambodia say it is driving sex workers underground, limiting access to sexual health services. Women who previously worked in brothels avoid the raids by using 'indirect' venues like karaoke bars, where clients take them off-site. This opens the door to heightened abuse and health risks for all involved. According to Tony Lisle, from UNAIDS, 'The crackdowns create significant difficulties for organizations working in HIV prevention to reach those who are most at risk from HIV infection effectively, particularly sex workers.'[138]

While the Cambodian drive is supposedly part of an anti-trafficking campaign, so far no traffickers have been arrested – only sex workers. Reports from Human Rights Watch confirm that the arrests do not locate trafficked women, and that non-trafficked women rounded up can be abused, raped, and thrown in prison. Some police and government officials use the law to commit crimes against the women.[139]

A US government diplomatic cable from 2006 confirms this is the case. It also shows that the situation has been known for some time. 'Targeting sex workers alone is not a viable solution to ridding Cambodia of prostitution nor is it particularly effective in addressing trafficking in persons. The fact that no pimps or brothel owners have been held responsible after the raids on nine brothels raises questions as to the government's motivations.'[140]

It is unlikely the government's actions will either catch traffickers or end consensual sex work, not least because an estimated one in three Cambodian men pays for sex. But they are driving sex workers underground and away from the healthcare they and their clients need. It seems likely continuing the crackdown will result in a higher rate of sexually transmitted infections.

There is a lot about human trafficking in the rest of the world that we don't know. Loads about trafficking in Europe and North America is misreported and misrepresented. What is clear is that anti-trafficking efforts that take a zero-tolerance approach to sex work do not catch traffickers and do not stop demand for sex work. Such schemes are rife with abuse and corruption, and put the health and safety of the public at risk. If we want to end trafficking of all kinds – a goal everyone agrees on – it's important to challenge assumptions about where and how it's happening.

Agenda Setters come in all shapes and guises. Some are clear about their intentions, others less so.

In Ireland, reports hyping the trafficking scare are also produced. For example, the Immigrant Council of Ireland (ICI), in 2009, released *Globalisation, Sex Trafficking and Prostitution: The Experiences of Migrant Women in Ireland*. It contains many of the same problems as its UK counterparts. But what is even more questionable than the content are the people producing it.

The Immigrant Council of Ireland promotes itself as an organisation giving support and advice to migrants and nothing immediately shouts 'religious agenda'. But, as it happens, there is a strong Catholic connection – with a controversial history.

The ICI was established by Sister Stanislaus Kennedy of the Religious Sisters of Charity, a Catholic order. The Catholic Church's position on prostitution is that it is a mortal sin and organisations with strong Catholic associations are at the forefront of attempts to criminalise prostitution in Ireland.

As it turns out, the Religious Sisters of Charity have been involved with 'rehabilitating' women in prostitution for a long time. They (along with three other orders) helped run the asylums for 'fallen women' known as Magdalene Laundries in Ireland, the last of which closed only in 1996.

The asylums were first established as short-term centres by evangelical Christians. After being appropriated by Catholic groups, the Magdalene movement transformed. It became a system of long-term institutions for unacceptable women. Their remit expanded to include not only former prostitutes, but also unwed mothers, developmentally challenged women, and abused girls. The tens of thousands of inmates were made to do hard physical labour, and endured a daily regime of enforced prayer and silence.

This came to a head in 1993 when one of the orders sold land to a developer. The remains of 155 inmates of the Magdalene Laundry were exhumed from an unmarked grave. Many former inmates of laundries have testified to sexual, psychological, and physical abuse that occurred within the asylums.

The Commission to Inquire into Child Abuse published the Ryan report in 2009. In the report, survivor accounts of Magdalene Laundries describe abuse that under most definitions amounted to slavery. Considering how recently the scandal broke, it's interesting to explore the background of some of the groups involved in government discourse on sex work and trafficking. What remains to be seen is what measures, exactly, they have in mind for trafficked women and sex workers.

There is evidence that trafficking and sex tourism are possibly more frequent in other parts of the world, and yet much time and attention is spent on a problem that can hardly be shown to even exist in Britain or the United States. The rights and self-determination of sex workers in the UK put them in a privileged position over many sex workers in the rest of the world, and yet the patronising concern that is expended on them would imply otherwise.

Does it matter? Yes, absolutely – when women's issues in the rest of the world lose out to the paranoid imaginations of the far right and the far left in this country.

Now, more than ever, people are questioning the ability of government and NGOs to address these issues. Money and time wasted on wild goose chases. Laws that prosecute the very people they're meant to help. Resources directed at a minority of victims, with more and more trafficked workers entering the non-sex labour market every day.

When asked directly, most people would acknowledge that the current approach to stopping trafficking has gone wrong. It rewards groups who pursue an extreme agenda. It embraces sloppy evidence and bad statistics. And a lot of people would recognise that lobbying by NGOs and charities is what makes it this way.

Enforcement of current laws should come before creation of new laws. Trafficking is already illegal. Breaking immigration laws is already illegal. Exploiting another person sexually for one's own gain is already illegal. The public, when asked, tends to agree that ensuring current laws are enforced is better than adding another layer of agencies, laws, and potential problems on top of the ones we already have. Victims of trafficking don't need more debates in Parliament or disorganised Keystone Kops schemes. They need the laws that already exist to protect them to be used the *right* way.

What is needed? Effective, efficient crime detection and policing of any abuses. What isn't? Special interest groups that claim all of the money to help only some of the victims. What we don't need is biased Constellation Makers turning out dodgy numbers to keep the focus on preconceptions rather than reality.

We also need greater understanding of the experiences of people who are trafficked, or are labelled as trafficked. Not all see themselves in that way, and as a result, a lot of the proposed solutions on offer are not relevant to their experiences. As someone who, by the way trafficking is counted, is supposedly 'trafficked', it feels like the diverse voices of people in migration and migratory labour (sex work or otherwise) are being ignored. Instead, others elect to speak for them. Who does this benefit?

There's a not-so-subtle undercurrent of sexism in the forced sex trafficking discussion. Time and again, women who say they in fact entered sex work knowingly have their experiences written off. This patronises women in ways that, frankly, would not happen to men. As researcher Laura Agustín comments, '[S]o entrenched is the idea of women as forming an essential part of home if not actually being it themselves that they are routinely denied the agency to undertake a migration.'[141] Women going to often underpaid, perhaps exploitative, work are painted universally as victims, regardless of their choices or options. Men going into often underpaid, perhaps exploitative work? Doing what society expects of them.

It's a funny kind of double standard, in which both sexes are subject to damaging assumptions. But it especially infantilises women, for whom low-paid domestic labour and sex work are frequently the only options if they have few skills and little education. Somehow, I doubt we'd ever be too up in arms about the welfare of men in the day-rate unskilled labour economy. This is an argument that is about the numbers, which is most of what this chapter addresses. But it also an argument that raises questions of how we define work, how we think about consent, and how exploitative all paid labour has the potential to be.

8

MYTH: Restricting and banning prostitution stops people from exchanging sex for money.

The first time I heard Michaela Hague's name was the day after she died.

It was my second year in Sheffield. I moved there in 2000 to start doctoral studies in the Forensic Pathology Department. During the first year, I lived in a converted church in the city centre, close to the department. The church had recently been renovated into a combination lecture hall and student flats. It was clean, modern, and comfortable.

St George's Church was also right in the middle of the red-light area.

The university literature had failed to mention that its Grade-II listed showpiece of student accommodation was also a popular landmark with Sheffield's streetwalkers and kerb crawlers. I figured it out quickly enough, though. I had no inkling at the time that, just four years later, I too would be working in the sex industry.

All things considered, it was not a bad place to live. For one thing, the furtive clients who came looking for sex rarely bothered us residents. The CCTV cameras, streetlights, and regular police cars cruising through the area added to a feeling of safety. And during the day, St George's looked respectable and sedate. As one of the very few people living in that area of the city, the sex trade didn't affect me; late-night student bars and noisy trams were more of a nuisance. I've lived in worse places, the sorts of places where drug deals happened in broad daylight and the sound of police – or worse, ambulance –

sirens was almost constant. St George's was nothing like that.

The area changed not long after, though. Perhaps under pressure from the university, which owned most of the buildings nearby. Or maybe the city fathers felt embarrassed by the show *Life of Grime*, which featured multiple episodes about places all within five minutes' walk of the church. Bollards appeared to stop cars circling round the neighbourhood. Women were moved off from the corners they usually worked. The street-based sex trade departed from the well-lit centre and relocated to the industrial areas around Corporation Street.

I moved out of St George's after a year. But I was still studying at the Medico-Legal Centre, where Sheffield's city mortuary shared space with the Forensic Pathology Department.

It was in that mortuary I saw what I would come to associate most strongly with the effects of driving the streetwalkers away from St George's.

The mortuary was a rectangular room, with parallel stations set up for performing autopsies. One particular morning I was called down to look at a postmortem that I still remember in excruciating detail. A young woman had been stabbed in a frenzied attack out past the dark underpasses of the Wicker, not far from Corporation Street. She lived long enough to give a partial description of her attacker, but died in hospital. The victim was just twenty-five years old. I had just turned twenty-six the night she died.

Michaela Hague was picked up by someone unknown, stabbed nineteen times, and left for dead. I remember her dark hair, the pathologist methodically recording the position and appearance of each place the knife entered. I remember the stuffed toy someone brought to the centre for her. Later I heard she had a seven-year-old son. Her killer has never been found.

Such a terrible, violent murder is only one tragedy. Many murders go unsolved every year. But the connection between what happened to Michaela and where she was working seemed clear to me. The more I learned, the more the effects of 'zero tolerance' policing seemed partly responsible for her untimely death. This would not have happened if she had been on the streets near St George's, with loads of walk-by traffic and well-lit corners. This crime could only have happened away from prying eyes, where anyone alerted to

Michaela's distress would not have been able to save her.

There is growing evidence that moving prostitutes into the darkened industrial outskirts of cities makes their lives more dangerous. Michaela Hague is just one victim of a policy that is more concerned with exploiting prostitution myths and preserving a façade of public order than it is about benefiting women.

Before discussing how current attitudes to sex work harm women, however, it might be instructive to take a little trip into our not-so-distant past.

The brothels that flourished in America's West in the late nineteenth century were remarkably liberating for the women who worked there. Prostitutes of that age enjoyed rights that mainstream feminism would access only much more slowly and decades later. In an era when women were barred from most jobs and had no ownership rights, sex workers made the highest wages of all American women and could even own property.

According to historian Ruth Rosen, the average brothel worker in those days earned from $1 to $5 per trick. Many earned more in a single night than women in other jobs could get in a week. She notes most prostitutes viewed their work as 'less oppressive than other survival strategies they might have chosen'.[142]

In the US in 1916, the average weekly wage for women in legitimate occupations was $6.67. Most women, of course, were not permitted to work and earned nothing at all. Skilled male tradesmen earned $20 per week. Prostitutes earned between $30 and $50 per week. Some women achieved financial comfort by marrying well, but with no property rights, rich wives actually possessed little of their own. By contrast, women choosing the sex trade could live well on their own terms, with their own money.[143]

A study of Virginia City, Nevada, shows that prostitutes in the 1860s boomtown were far from naïve 'white slaves'. 'From the age data on prostitutes, it is clear that they were old enough to realize the nature of their behavior and also old enough to have married had they so desired, for this was an area with many unattached men. Thus we conclude that these were professional women intent on economic success,' wrote historians George Blackburn and Sherman Ricards.[144]

The average age of a prostitute in the Old West was twenty-three.

Timothy Gilfoyle wrote about how during the nineteenth century 'an affluent, but migratory, class of prostitutes flourished.' A class that questioned the wisdom of working in factories, when sex work was better paid, and arguably safer. One prostitute of the time is quoted: 'Do you suppose I am going back to earn five or six dollars a week in a factory, and at that, never have a cent of it to spend for myself, when I can earn that amount any night, and often much more?'[145]

Brothel madams were prominent citizens of their communities and funded public works projects throughout the West. In Denver, madam Jennie Rogers paid for water services to the city. 'Diamond Jessie' Hayman gave food and clothing to thousands left homeless by San Francisco's devastating 1906 earthquake. Lou Graham of Seattle, 'Queen of the Lava Beds', helped fund the city's public school system. Anna Wilson, 'Queen of the Omaha Underworld', bequeathed her mansion to the city in her will. It became the region's first emergency hospital and infectious disease clinic.

There were few more powerful black women in that time than Mary Ellen 'Mammy' Pleasant. Pleasant escaped indentured servitude and became a successful madam in San Francisco. She worked with the Underground Railroad, moving people trapped in slave states to free territory, and was a financial supporter of revolutionary abolitionist John Brown. As well as investing in mining stock and making loans to the city's elite, Pleasant earned the moniker 'the mother of human rights in California' after filing a lawsuit to desegregate San Francisco's streetcars.

According to research by Paula Petrik, 60 per cent of prostitutes in Helena, Montana, in the 1860s 'reported either personal wealth or property or both'. Prostitutes' average monthly income there was $233 – far higher than that of skilled tradesmen who earned $90 and 'white collar' men making $125 per month. The red-light district in Helena was (according to Petrik) 'women's business grounded in women's property and capital'.[146]

There were many court cases in which prostitutes challenged men who assaulted or robbed them, and frequently with positive results. In half of such cases, 'the judge or jury found for the female complainants'. A pretty successful ratio, even by today's standards. And blind eyes were turned where and when it was sensible to do so: there was 'a singular lack of legal and judicial concern with sexual commerce ... [O]fficers of the law arrested no women for prostitution or keeping a disorderly house before 1886, even though the police court was located in the red-light district.'

It wasn't only about the money. Madams also supplied birth control, legal assistance, and accommodation. They provided healthcare decades before other employers did. While women in the general population had little recourse against violence, even in cases of marital rape, madams enlisted police and bodyguards to protect their employees.

Fiction has an outsize influence not only on perceptions of trafficking, but also on feelings about prostitution. Of the many depictions of prostitution in recent UK television dramas, only one is based directly on a nonfiction memoir of prostitution – and it is widely accused of glamorising sex work by presenting a protagonist who is neither drug-addicted nor abused. Yes, of course I'm referring to *Secret Diary of a Call Girl*.

Most other media depictions of prostitution, however, rely on stereotypes of streetwalkers and other sex workers having chaotic, desperate lives. Even the Home Office supports this distortion. Until recently it had a website which claimed: 'Most women involved in street-based prostitution are not there through choice ... Nearly all prostitutes are addicted to drugs or alcohol. Many of them have been trafficked into the country by criminals, and are held against their will. Many were abused as children, and many are homeless.'[147] There were no sources given for these statements – for the simple fact that they are wrong.

As sex educator and ex-sex worker Carol Queen notes in *Real Live Nude Girls*, 'A weapon consistently used against the marginalized is ... insidious myth-making, leading outsiders to believe things about individuals, based on their group status, that may not be true.'[148]

This reliance on fiction over truth influences how information is obtained and distributed. Lamenting the narrow focus of most research, Laura Agustín notes, '[T]he focus is usually on personal motivations, the morality of the buying-and-selling relationship, stigma, violence and disease prevention.'[149] Unfortunately, those focused on opposing sex work very often come across as opposed to sex workers themselves, rather than the work as such. Preconceived opinions are seldom challenged.

The reality of prostitution is rarely the *Pretty Woman* ending, but it's also seldom as grim as *Band of Gold*. It's incredibly diverse, attracting all kinds of people with all kinds of motivations and ways of working in the business.

When researchers allow sex workers to tell their experiences in a way that does not prejudge the outcome, the results reveal things that are well known to those in the work, but still news to people on the outside. A 2009 study polling sex workers is an excellent case in point. *Beyond Gender: An examination of exploitation in sex work* by Suzanne Jenkins of Keele University revealed the results of detailed interviews with 440 sex workers.[150] Not simply street-based women, either, but women, men, and transgendered sex workers in all areas of the business. Over half were from the UK; the rest were based in Western Europe, North America, Australia, and New Zealand.

The results turn almost everything we think we know about sex work on its head.

Is paid sex all about clients dominating sex workers? No. Less than 7 per cent of the women interviewed thought that paying for sex gives the client power over the escort; 26.2 per cent thought paying makes clients vulnerable; while the majority, 54.5 per cent, said that 'Commercial sexual transactions are relationships of equality.'

People generally think that clients get whatever they want from sex workers, abusing and taking advantage of them. But when asked, 'In your escort interactions who normally takes overall control of the encounter?' 77 per cent said they always or they usually did, 22.3 per cent said it varies, and only 0.7 per cent said the client decides.

Sex work is often characterised as brutal, with abuse a commonplace and even usual outcome. But when asked if they have ever felt physically threatened, only 25 per cent of women and 18.7 per cent of men said yes; 77 per cent of women said they felt clients treated them respectfully; the same percentage said they respected their clients.

When asked, 'How much longer do you plan to do escort work for?', 'I have no plans to stop escort work' was joint first choice of answer for women along with 'one to five more years' (both receiving 35.3 per cent). Only 3.2 per cent said they planned to stop in less than three months. In many ways, this reflects a pragmatism familiar to anyone with a more 'traditional' career.

Sex workers are often stereotyped as very young and naïve, unaware of the dangers of the choices they are making. But the age data do not suggest the field is populated with teenage runaways and naïve youngsters. Almost 85 per cent of the women were aged 26 or older, and 19 per cent of them were over 40.

Sex work is frequently assumed to be a choice suitable only for the uneducated. But 35.3 per cent of the men and 32.9 per cent of the women had degrees, and over 18 per cent of the total held postgraduate qualifications. Only 6.5 per cent had no formal educational qualifications.

When you compare these statistics to the general population of the UK, they compare very favourably. Overall, only 20 per cent of adults of all ages have degrees, rather lower than the respondents in this sex work study. But with only a handful of sex workers over retirement age, they skew slightly younger than all adults, so it is more suitable to compare this group to younger people. Data from 2008 shows that 35 per cent of young British people now attain degrees: almost identical to the proportion among sex workers.[151] The proportion of all Britons under age 40 with no formal educational qualifications at all, at 8 per cent, is rather higher than it is in sex workers.[152]

The balance between risk and reward is something people address all the time. Whether one picks a career as a deep-sea fisherman or as a call girl, the potential income and danger are well publicised, and yet people sign up willingly. This is a choice everyone has the right to make for him- or herself.

When asked what things they like about the work, two in three respondents in the Keele study reported 'like meeting people'; 75 per cent of women and 50 per cent of men reported 'flexibility of working hours' as an aspect they enjoy; 72 per cent of women cited 'independence'. Jenkins noted: 'An appreciation of flexible working hours and independence were factors that were valuable to women generally, not only mothers. The benefits of greater independence and flexible working hours were not just about the demands of parenting – they were often about time provided for other, non parenting-related pursuits.'

This was certainly true in my case: the short hours of work I performed as a call girl left ample time to look for science jobs, finish writing my doctoral thesis, and participate in a demanding sport at a high level. Juggling those things with a job as a waitress or behind a bar not only wouldn't have paid the bills, it wouldn't have left time to pursue a professional career. It can be damned hard to better yourself if you're too tired to think about anything but where the next month's rent is coming from.

When discussing these issues, however, one often runs up against people who are convinced that the picture is very different. Sometimes they even quote studies. But are these studies good sources of data? Let's consider the interim report of Eaves for Women and London South Bank University PE:ER Project (Prostitution Exiting: Engaging through Research) that came out in May 2011.

The first and most striking problem with the report? The sample they've recruited is not representative of UK sex workers overall. For one thing, it only surveys female sex workers.

That alone is enough reason to be sceptical of the results, because they don't make it clear men and transgender people are excluded. While women represent the majority of UK sex workers, they are by no means all. But those devoting their efforts to the 'rescue' of sex workers love to focus on women. Organisations like Eaves don't count and don't cater for male and transgender sex workers.

The second problem is that the types of sex workers they survey are not representative. It's tough to get exact numbers, but it's estimated that street-based workers only account for 5–20 per cent of all sex work. In the Eaves report, streetwalkers comprise 62.3 per cent of the respondents. Why is this a problem? Because in assessing such issues as drug use and abuse, they report overall averages of their sample and extrapolate to sex workers in the country as a whole. Their averages will be skewed, heavily, by not having a representative sample. There is no correction made in the data for this difference between their chosen sample and the sex worker population at large.

Another way in which the results are distorted is by classifying 6.1 per cent of respondents as 'trafficked'. Again, this is far higher than is true in the UK as a whole. And that's not even considering the problem of what definition of 'trafficked' they're using.

As a former statistician dealing with population-based data, I know that one of the most important criteria for an acceptable study is to make sure the sampled population reflects the status of the population as a whole. If this is not done, the results are not reliable.

The work by Suzanne Jenkins at Keele contained responses from 29 men (26.6 per cent of respondents) and 8 per cent of her respondents were transgender. This certainly is similar to my own experience. When I worked as an escort, there were about twenty girls represented by the agency, and four men.

The second problem with the PE:ER Project report is how respondents were found: the majority, 88.5 per cent, were recruited through support services. Who accesses support services? People who need help, of course. It would be a little like surveying a divorce court and claiming the results were representative of all married couples!

What claims does the PE:ER Project make? The rate of drug dependency in the women working on the streets was 71.8 per cent. That in itself is interesting, since it is widely assumed that all street sex workers are drug addicts, and seven in ten is a long way from 'all'. But it is still very high. Notably, in their numbers about sex workers based off the streets, the rates plummet to less than a third. It seems reasonable to assume, since they only recruited through support services, that the reality is that a lot less than 70 per cent of street-based workers are addicts, and that a lot less than 30 per cent of the off-street workers are. But the potential gulf between the people they queried and sex workers as a whole is never addressed.

There are other interesting questions raised by their numbers that they don't bother to examine. For instance, the fact that drug dependency in off-street sex workers is half what it is for those on the streets suggests that it might be problems with addiction that influence where sex workers end up, not the other way round. The report seems to assume that sex work causes addiction, without considering that the causal relationship could easily be the other way round.

The study also reports that an additional one in ten (10.5 per cent) of the women were using drugs on a recreational level. That sounds like a lot. But is it? No comparisons are made with the general population anywhere in the report. In fact, this percentage is comparable with the UK in general. The British Crime Survey estimates 12 per cent of respondents in England and Wales and 9 per cent in Scotland are recreational drug users – among students, the percentages of recreational drug use are even higher.[153]

So many of the beliefs repeated about prostitution are wrong, easily disproven ... and believed with almost religious fervour. Ever hear the one that claims, 'seventy-five per cent of women in prostitution become involved when they are under the age of eighteen'? Let's look at the data. It turns out that in the UK, the breakdown is average age of twenty-one for streetwalkers, twenty-five for off-street and agency escorts, and nearly thirty-two for sauna sex workers.[154] So, for the '75 per cent' claim to be even plausible, some interesting data manipulation needs to have happened. The number would be more likely to be accurate if the majority of sex workers were streetwalkers. But as this isn't the case, it must be that the number comes from studies of limited size that only looked at young streetwalkers, and extrapolated this to prostitution in general.

Another common claim is that 45 per cent of prostitutes report childhood sexual abuse and 85 per cent childhood physical abuse. These figures derive from a paper on streetwalkers which was commissioned as part of a crime reduction programme.[155] It involved a handful of interviews with women in sex work who were contacted in conjunction with drop-in centres. Did it compare these data against comparable, non-sex work people accessing similar services? Was there a control population? No. In other words, the results are statistically pointless.

Speaking of which, you can tell a lot about a study by who is recruited to give input. In that particular study, tables show that the survey respondents included 872 'local community members', 139 'project staff' (including police), and fewer than 40 people actually involved in sex work. Of which none were men.

Studies that focus exclusively on streetwalkers are widely relied on by anti-prostitution writers. The reason why these studies are not representative as they claim is because the lives of many streetwalkers are so much more chaotic than the lives of the majority of prostitutes.

A 2005 study by Ronald Weitzer of George Washington University highlights a number of these differences.[156] It found that escorts saw their work positively, while the brothel girls were merely satisfied and streetwalkers were mainly dissatisfied. It found that 97 per cent of escorts surveyed reported an increase in self-esteem after they started sex work, compared with 50 per cent of Nevada brothel workers and 8 per cent of streetwalkers. Other studies from elsewhere in the world confirm this – a Dutch study from 2004 showed similar results.[157] An earlier study from the US found that 75 per cent of escorts felt that their lives had improved since starting sex work, 25 per cent reported no change. No respondents said their lives were worse.[158] An Australian study found that half of all prostitutes considered their work as a 'major source of satisfaction' in their lives; 70 per cent said they would choose sex work again if they had their lives to live over.[159]

The most recent push to eliminate street prostitution really took off in the 1990s. The Labour party was inspired by the highly publicised 'cleanup' of Times Square in New York City by mayor Rudy Giuliani. Shadow Home Secretary Jack Straw recommended 'reclaiming the streets for the law-abiding citizen', with Shadow Leader Tony Blair endorsing 'Operation Zero Tolerance'. Once in government, Labour continued to focus on an approach to crime reduction that aggressively cracked down on visible exchange of money for sex.[160]

While having sex for money is legal, soliciting and loitering are not. As a result, prostitution crackdowns overwhelmingly target streetwalkers. While it's hard to come by exact numbers, evidence shows streetwalkers only account for 5–20 per cent of all prostitutes – the remaining 80–95 per cent work elsewhere, such as in brothels, in massage parlours, or as call girls.[161]

It's widely assumed that the presence of streetwalking, brothels, and the like promotes crime. Streetwalking appears to happen more often in dodgy areas. But one of the problems with data is teasing out the cause from the effect. In other words, is prostitution something that encourages local crime, or do streetwalkers happen to work in areas in which higher crime rates already exist?

You might expect the government to be interested in which came first in this chicken-or-egg situation but, by and large, they are not. Consider the Home Office document *Kerb-Crawling, Prostitution and Multi-Agency Policing*.[162] The report looks at a police crackdown in Finsbury Park, London. Its very first sentence states, 'When centred upon residential areas, street prostitution and kerb-crawling can significantly reduce the quality of life enjoyed by a local population.'

Because the idea of 'significance' has numerical and statistical connotations, you should expect any document that claims to be fact-based and invokes the idea of significance to be prepared to back it up with numbers. I'm afraid if you're going to say something has been 'significantly' reduced, then you're going to have to quantify that.

Does this paper do so? The answer, predictably enough, is no. They do trot out a few polls, though. A poll estimates 89 per cent of residents think prostitution is a 'major problem', but that means nothing in terms of real increase in crime and real effects on the area.

Does prostitution 'significantly' affect crime? No idea. Do people feel it does? Yes – but that's not the same thing. Popular perception is a strange thing, and not the same as reality. For example, 61 per cent of Americans believe the world was created in seven days. That's not the same thing as there being evidence of it happening. It's not even the same as there being a 'significant' chance that it happened.

The paper states, 'Tackling kerb-crawling and street prostitution in an area leads to its displacement or deflection to alternative sites.' Now that is interesting. It could imply that the authors are concerned about the welfare of sex workers who are moved on. After all, the welfare of those involved is surely as important as homeowners' feelings, right?

Ah, no. '[A]lthough there was some evidence of displacement, it was to areas such as the nearby shopping streets, which residents found less objectionable.'

In other words, it is house prices and the appearance of propriety the Finsbury Park effort was bothered about, not sex workers' safety and health. The only result desired – and obtained – was that the streetwalkers moved to a less populated area. And it is a result that puts them at higher risk of attack.

Contrary to popular belief, streetwalkers don't just jump into any car. That would be, even in a job people think of as inherently dangerous, an unacceptable level of risk. In fact, streetwalkers often get together to discuss strategies for reducing harm. They do this by sharing number plates and descriptions of dodgy kerb crawlers, vetting clients, and only going to places they know. Outreach services like drop-in centres and night vans also help this effort, keeping 'ugly mugs' books and being a valuable point of contact. Streetwalkers perform a balancing act between maximising client exposure, while still avoiding potential harm.

When police and vigilante residents displace sex workers, women have a new balancing act to negotiate – one that puts them at a disadvantage. This is something that has happened time and again in Britain.

The once well-established red-light area of Balsall Heath in Birmingham, where prostitutes sat in the windows of flats along Cheddar Road, started to be targeted in the 1990s by the Muslim community. Groups of men went after the women, both while they were working and when they weren't. It was a campaign of harassment meant to drive the red lights away for good.

Harassment forces sex workers to get into clients' cars quickly, and possibly be unable to avoid dangerous kerb crawlers. When vigilantes and police roam the pavements, sex workers wait until the wee hours to come out, making them more isolated and vulnerable to harm.[163]

In the end, those actions did not improve sex workers' lives. Prostitutes left Balsall Heath alright, but not for a different kind of work. They simply relocated, many going two miles away to Edgbaston, and the cycle began anew.

Such an approach can also result in a transfer of activity from streetwalking to other ways of obtaining money. High-profile crackdown results in repeated arrests, which translate to fines that sex workers, now burdened with criminal records, are unable to pay except by more prostitution or by fraud, shoplifting, and dealing drugs.[164]

Take Aberdeen, for instance. From 2001 onwards, the city had an established tolerance zone for sex workers around the harbour. That ended with passage of the Prostitution (Public Places) (Scotland) Act in 2007. In the following months, the city centre experienced an influx of streetwalkers and an increase in petty crimes.

Quay Services, which operates a drop-in centre for streetwalkers, reported that sex workers became more afraid to seek assistance, and the number of women coming to the centre dropped to 'just a handful'.[165] There was also evidence that displacing sex workers led to more activity in the sex trade, not less – convictions for solicitation tripled.[166] This kind of 'crime shuffling' takes prostitution out of one area and dumps it on another. It only resembles an improvement if you fail to look at the full picture.

High reoffending rates among some sex workers are at least partly due to the fact that people who have ever broken the law are seen as only criminals, no matter what they do next. It's difficult to function in the straight world with a record. All the po-faced feminism in the world is not going to change the fact that many people are (understandably) reluctant to hire someone with a criminal past. In some places, such as some US states, being convicted of soliciting sex puts you on the sex offenders' register as well. Illinois, for instance, lists 'public indecency' and 'indecent solicitation of an adult' as worthy of sex offender status.

It's for these reasons I believe the opponents of legal sex work endorse policies that make a person's life outcomes narrower, harder, and more punitive than is ever necessary. The mumbled slogans about 'turning lives around' is a red herring when all the drop-in centres in the world won't get you a legitimate job. There's so much emphasis put on shelters, transitions, and all the rest of it: then what? The spiral of hopelessness is simply not broken by pat answers and vote-winning 'tough on crime' nonsense.

Even groups who say their priority is reducing violence towards women still back a strategy of criminalisation that puts sex workers in danger. The Poppy Project, in its response to the Home Office's *Paying the Price* consultation on prostitution, reiterated that its agenda was to continue to support the criminalisation of clients of sex workers and offences not directly associated with prostitution but commonly associated with it.

Policies that address prostitution only in terms of crime have a knock-on effect on how its participants are viewed by the public. If someone who has ever worked on the streets is murdered, her death is reported in the media not as 'woman killed', but as 'prostitute killed'. Over and again much is made in the press of how isolated street-walkers are, the problems they have, their chaotic lives.

In everything I ever read about Michaela Hague in Sheffield, she was described as a good friend, a caring mother, and a nice person. It's unlikely Michaela would have defined herself solely as a prostitute. Yet, just for having ever accepted money for sex, laws are written that treat the rights of sex workers as different from those of 'normal' people. Fiction, news, and ideology all spend a lot of time emphasising that it's usual, and even acceptable, to think of these people as inherently different from others. Many organisations accept money and instead of helping people, support their criminalisation.

Many people who have no first-hand knowledge of what sex work is like claim to be telling the 'real' story of prostitution, and shout down anyone who disagrees. It is as if simply by having taken money for sex, you are rendered incapable of speaking for yourself. To be, as I am, a former sex worker with anything to say that isn't 100 per cent negative about prostitution, is to be written off, disregarded, and ridiculed by people who imagine their preconceptions somehow carry more weight than my actual lived experience.

We continually hear how prostitution is dangerous, and death all but guaranteed. Poor handling of investigations like Peter Sutcliffe's show how, at least in the past, police have sometimes been less than perfectly careful when investigating the murders of prostitutes. So, when a serial killer emerges who is targeting sex workers, few are surprised.

Violence against sex workers is rarely reported because, seriously, since when have the police ever been on the side of sex workers? On a day-to-day basis, sex workers are more likely to have a negative encounter with police than they are with a client.

Perhaps, rather than assuming these women are targeted because they are prostitutes, we should consider that they may be targeted because of the message society is sending about their value as humans. Gary Ridgway, also known as the Green River Killer, murdered forty-eight women in America in the early 1980s. He later talked about why most of his victims were streetwalkers: 'I picked prostitutes as victims because they were easy to pick up without being noticed. I knew they would not be reported missing right away and might never be reported missing. I thought I could kill as many of them as I wanted without getting caught.' [167]

It wasn't the commercial sex angle that was attractive to him, but the convenience. Many such killers are opportunists; they not only target shamed outsiders like prostitutes, but also hitchhikers and people travelling alone. People whose whereabouts are not exactly known at any given time. And yet no one would endorse a law criminalising solo travel under the rubric of 'protecting' holidaymakers – that would be ludicrous.

The mental health problems associated with outsider status are well known. Social isolation increases the risk of violence, blackmail, and coercion. Stigma and fear of humiliation and prosecution exacerbates any existing mental health issues. The current policy therefore is responsible for many of the mental health issues associated with sex work.

Not all is negative. There are some hopeful and encouraging things going on that actually could benefit sex workers and reduce their exposure to harm. In Liverpool, police adopted a policy that recognises violence against sex workers as a hate crime. The result is that they can approach the police and know that violence against them will be taken seriously. This has led to a dramatic increase in prosecutions and a decline in assaults. But it's a model that has yet to be picked up anywhere else.

Perhaps the greatest danger to prostitutes comes when culture promotes the idea that sex workers are less than fully protected by the law. It's a reality Gary Ridgway knew and exploited, like many serial killers before and since. And when prostitutes are attacked, it adds fuel to the fire of prohibitionists who believe making sex work illegal and shifting it to industrial parks will somehow solve the problem. Chicken, meet egg.

The American West may loom large in our collective imaginations, but in reality it did not last very long at all. In the years following the US Civil War, the federal government started preparing western territories to become fully fledged states. Lawmaking procedures and regional government were standardised. As well as bringing in a considerable amount of red tape, this also helped pave the way for a population boom.

Increased migration brought more families, more churches, and a greater influence of prudishness to the Wild West. As family settlements began to overtake saloons, new arrivals were shocked by what they encountered. The inevitable result was social pressure to change the laws in areas that had until then tolerated prostitution. In 1890, an alliance of social reformers pressured the US Congress to form a national crime commission to investigate the sex trade. When Congress refused, the social reformers started their own.

The reports produced by these 'vice committees' were weapons in the war against prostitution. They were cited in forty-three cities' bans on the sex trade. The reports claimed to be objective, yet contained material that was strong-armed from sex workers and used to blackmail political opponents. Social purity movements forced 'soiled doves' into workhouses to 'rehabilitate' them. Young women deemed to be at risk were forcibly removed from their homes. With a combination of dodgy methods and underhand tactics, opponents of prostitution transformed their morality crusades into real political power.

Reports that are written today – such as the *Paying the Price* consultation by the Home Office, or any of a number of self-published reports written by NGOs such as Eaves – are designed precisely to sway government policy and public opinion to fall in line with their agendas.

Back in the nineteenth and early twentieth centuries, eugenicists believed that inherited degeneracy and 'feeble-mindedness' caused women to enter prostitution. Today, the party line is that prostitutes were sexually abused as children, and are emotionally unstable, or otherwise incapable of making their own decisions. Therefore it is up to what Laura Agustín has termed the 'rescue industry' to step in.

The assumption that prostitution is a damaging occupation undertaken only by damaged people underpins manipulated reports from the nineteenth century to today. The bias tends towards certain methods of conducting studies and certain ways of reporting the results. Everything is affected from who is chosen to interview, to how questionnaire content is written. If the *a priori* assumption is that prostitution is dreadful, then it is unsurprising when the results of a study return a picture that is unsavoury.

The recent writings of Melissa Farley are typical of the output. Farley is a director of a non-profit organisation called Prostitution Research and Education based in San Francisco. She has a handful of papers and self-published books that are commonly quoted in arguments against legalising prostitution. In terms of influence, she's a classic Constellation Maker, funding and publishing her own research, then broadcasting the results through an Evangelising organisation she founded herself.

In 'Prostitution and trafficking in Nevada: making the connections', Farley claimed 90 per cent of sex workers 'wish they could get out'. But prostitution in Nevada is illegal, except for the highly regulated 'pussy penitentiary' brothels in rural counties where the women are often compelled to work long shifts and multiple weeks without days off, and where they are forbidden even to bring their own cars to the compounds. So, the only people she interviewed were by definition either working illegally, or confined to bunker-like workplaces far from home. It's not representative of prostitution in general, and she does not include control groups or interviews with other sex workers anywhere.

There's also the question of whether such job dissatisfaction is confined to sex work. As it happens, across all employment sectors, less than 40 per cent of under-25s are satisfied with their work.[168] Even respectable jobs like teaching have problems, with 40 per cent of qualified UK teachers leaving due to stress and unhappiness within two years.[169] Job dissatisfaction is not unique to sex work, and a projected 10 per cent satisfaction rate (in other words, 90 per cent of employees wishing they could get out) in unskilled work is common. Though, of course, there actually are studies showing far higher rates of job satisfaction in sex workers to contrast with the grim picture engineered in her study. Farley doesn't mention any of them.

One of Farley's other papers, reporting on post-traumatic stress disorder in prostitutes, demonstrates a host of problems. It recruited respondents found at drug abuse drop-in centres, collecting data from a pool of people one would expect to have higher rates of mental trauma than even other sex workers. Again, there was no control population with other sex workers or other non-sex workers.[170] Studies of PTSD in sex workers have been heavily criticised both for their sources of funding (the neo-conservative Bush administration in the US) and for being carried out by people who do not have the appropriate qualifications.[171]

The criticism has gained momentum. In September 2011, Dr Calum Bennachie filed a complaint with the American Psychology Association asking that they rescind the membership of Melissa Farley.

In the complaint, Dr Bennachie lists a number of reasons for doing so.[172] The reasons include factual errors in some of her papers that appear to be misleading. Also mentioned is Farley's apparent failure to seek ethical approval from the New Zealand Psychological Society (NZPsS). In many countries, when doing research that involves the participation of specific people or in which individuals could be identified from their answers, such approval must always be sought before research begins. It's not a fun part of being a researcher – I once spent nine months of a twelve-month grant just preparing and processing ethics-related paperwork – but it is necessary. Bennachie also notes that 'she claimed to be able to diagnose sex workers as having post-traumatic stress disorder, despite using a flawed questionnaire, and not doing in-depth interviews.'

If these complaints are true, and the work is indeed unethical, it possibly breaches sections 5.01 and 8.10 of the APA's Code of Ethics. With so many anti-sex-work writers and activists not only referencing her work, but also consulting her as an expert in these topics, it's an accusation that certainly merits a deeper look. The people who work with human subjects, particularly in psychology and particularly where they are targeting potentially at-risk populations for their data, should definitely be scrutinised on these kinds of claims.

Such examples show how prostitution is a hard issue for feminists to address. Many continue to equate prostitution with violence against women with little or no supporting data. For instance, Julie Bindel wrote in 2010, 'Prostitution is both the cause and consequence of inequality between men and women'[173] (a logical impossibility if ever there was one). Funny, because I can think of plenty of places where prostitution is illegal but inequality between men and women is worse than in the UK. Iran, for instance. Saudi Arabia. Afghanistan. Imagining that criminalising prostitution levels the playing field between men and women is ludicrous.

Even strident anti-sex-work writers like Julie Bindel can sometimes seem confused about whether the approach they endorse actually works. In a 2003 article, she even appears to admit – in a roundabout sort of way – that making sex work illegal might do more harm than good. In a lengthy piece on female sex tourists in the Dominican Republic, which does little to demonise the white, middle-class women paying for West Indian men, she notes: 'There are obvious differences between female and male sex tourism ... they [are not] vulnerable to criminalisation, unlike female prostitutes whose activities are illegal.'[174] I tell you my gob was well and truly smacked to think that Bindel herself might actually be suggesting that criminalisation does, indeed, have a part in making sex workers vulnerable.

Others demonstrate a naïvety about economic reality that is almost touching in its innocence. Catherine Redfern writes of prostitution that '[n]o one should be forced to do any kind of work that they really don't want to do, simply to survive.'[175] Which is rather amazing given that the vast majority of all waged work is probably done for exactly that reason. How many people does she reckon restocking the shelves in supermarkets are there because it's what they always dreamed of doing?

Most people have to work to earn a living. In my experience, having sex for money was far better than the long, long list of low-paid, exploitative, going-nowhere jobs I had as a student. I worked briefly as a charity mugger, which was infinitely more depressing. I worked in a call centre, being yelled at and hung up on by literally thousands of people. I was taken advantage of and underpaid in countless retail jobs and several research ones. Never once did I experience in sex work the dehumanisation that I experienced daily in many of those other jobs (and often for far less pay). And my experience of that is far from unique.

Sex work is the only profession in which commentators assume you must hate the thing you do in order to take money for it. That would be like accusing Gordon Ramsay of hating food. Sure, there are probably a lot of people working in fast food who barely tolerate their jobs, but no one assumes that's a condition of employment. Most long-term career sex workers I know don't hate sex and don't hate their jobs.

Sex work is infinitely more complex, and approaching it under the umbrella of assuming all sex workers are streetwalkers is a problem. Heck, assuming all streetwalkers are the same is a problem. 'Being a streetwalker' is not a discrete outcome of a single experience.

Let's say that, included among sex workers on the street, there are:

- people who are in large amounts of debt they can't pay off
- people who are homeless or vulnerably housed

- people with mental health issues or addictions that make it difficult to be hired, or fulfil the demands of most kinds of waged work
- people with criminal records, who find it difficult to get jobs
- people who have been marginalised by the system, such as having been raised in care, and attaining adulthood without a good support system
- people whose health drove them onto the street, and who have no way out
- people who simply want to do this work (this may be a small number, but it's intellectually dishonest to say it doesn't exist)
- and many more.

There are a lot of people, of course, who would look at that list and write off every category on it as not deserving of support. I'm going to make the assumption that readers progressing past this point don't believe that.

Each of these groups has different needs. There are some solutions that overlap, but others that would only be suitable for one group. Any programme that claims to serve the needs of this population must provide the essentials of a quality of life as well as the stepping stones to get out of prostitution if they choose to take them. It must also accept that some people may not choose to take those steps.

Over and again, when sex workers are asked why they do the job, the answers revolve around two issues: money and time. Without a sea change in the ways people have access to money and time, there will always be prostitution. Always.

Further, even if these issues are addressed, there are still people who will choose to do sex work. Some among those will take up its most visible and dangerous forms. This is an uncomfortable truth about sex work, one that is written off. Again and again, actual sex workers with actual experience in the business who do not paint the work as universally awful or say they would do it again are told they have 'false consciousness' or are 'fake' and 'lying'. Fine, whatever. Attributing your assumptions to someone else's thought process is a dangerous game to play, but we all do it sometimes.

It's when the people saying those things are also affiliated with, or supporting, the 'rescue industry' that I have a problem. How is it possible to offer comprehensive assistance that has a real outcome to people you think are deluded or lying? How is it possible to offer compassionate support to people you belittle? The short and obvious answer is that it isn't. It's like becoming a pharmacist when you really believe in homeopathy. The two are not compatible.

Women in danger, women who can't defend themselves, women who hate themselves and their lives ... the arguments made by feminist opponents of sex work bear surprising similarities to those made by social conservatives of the nineteenth century. The result? An atmosphere in which both the far left and the far right claim to know better than women themselves do. In these analyses there are no shades of grey.

Labelling sex workers as victims is dangerous ground for anyone who claims to be in favour of women's equality. It presents them as all the same and denies them a voice in the debate. Also, many who advocate eliminating prostitution have neither worked in it nor have they conducted peer-reviewed research in it. As supposed experts, their exposure to the topic is no more in-depth than that of anyone else who watches movies or reads the paper.

The way the sex work issue has been handled elsewhere can give us useful insights into what does, and does not, work. The legalisation of prostitution in New Zealand is one such example.

As both Europe and the US embraced colonialism, venturing into unknown territory didn't just mean opening supply routes around the globe. For many indigenous people, first contact with Europeans also brought exposure to the sex trade. As in the American West, there was money to be made from men who rarely travelled with female company. New Zealand was no different.[176]

By the nineteenth century, in New Zealand, as in most British dependencies, pressure was exacted to pass the Contagious Diseases Act, and to heavily prosecute the 'social evil'. But after the Massage Parlours Act in 1978 allowed massage as a de facto cover for indoor prostitution, lobby groups in New Zealand began to push for legalisation of sex work across the board.

In 2003, New Zealand opted to overturn their laws that criminalised prostitution in favour of regulation. The people most visibly affected by the law were streetwalkers in larger cities like Auckland, where in 2003 about 360 girls were estimated by police to be working. Streetwalkers represent about 11 per cent of the total number of prostitutes in the country.[177]

Suddenly, the world's focus was on New Zealand: would legalisation change the sex trade there, and if so, how? Would it benefit the women, or harm them? What would it do to neighbourhoods, to tourism, to the country's international image?

An evaluation released several years later showed that the number of sex workers changed very little – and in some places, the numbers of them on the streets actually decreased – compared to before sex work was legal. In Auckland, the estimated number of girls working the streets decreased significantly, from 360 to 106. People working in massage parlours and other establishments expressed a desire to stay in the work because of the financial rewards.[178]

However, the report came under fire from the usual suspects. Melissa Farley in particular attacked the evaluation, saying that the numbers actually increased.[179] She provided no evidence to support her claim. This is unsurprising since the report used verifiable numbers obtained through reliable channels and would be difficult to challenge with any credibility. The numbers in the official evaluation came from police estimates and actual headcounts, which are straightforward since New Zealand cities are rather small.

Farley also claimed that the UN found evidence for trafficking and child prostitution in New Zealand after 2003 – but does she establish a causal link between trafficking and the law change? No. Is there discussion of what the situation may have been before 2003? No. As we have seen previously, correlation does not prove causation ... and Farley's paper does not even give any evidence of increase in trafficking.

In 2010, a book was published that included interviews with over 700 sex workers in New Zealand.[180] The number of interviews represents almost 12 per cent of the estimated 5932 prostitutes in the country, a far higher proportion than in virtually any other qualitative study of sex workers ever conducted. It concluded that the majority entered and stayed in the sex trade for financial reasons, that they felt the new laws gave them more protection, and that the result was positive changes overall for safety and health.

Many of the prostitutes reported that social stigma was still a problem, but that as a result of the legislation they had become more willing (and able) to report crimes to the police. Which surely represents a victory for women's safety.

On the other side of the world, in Sweden, a law was passed in 1999 – *sexköpslagen* – that criminalised the buyers (but not the providers) of sex. Norway and Iceland adopted similar laws in 2009. Even before the Swedish government's own evaluation in 2010 of whether the law had been a success, the UK's anti-sex-work concerns were claiming it was the panacea Britain needed.

Was it? The evaluation, released in July 2010, relied heavily on a scattering of data about street prostitution, as other sex trade activities have become, presumably, far harder to identify as a result of *sexköpslagen*. It also included data from – wait for it – seven active sex workers and seven former sex workers, a rather small sample by anyone's standards. The evaluation compared the same time period to streetwalking activity in Denmark, where there is no such law. But those data came from a Copenhagen NGO whose numbers claimed the number of streetwalkers in Denmark was about six times higher than it actually is.[181]

The bulk of the analysis focused instead on reiterating ideological arguments about why prostitution was bad. But as to any actual information … it's severely lacking. The report has next to nothing about Swedes accessing sex services using the internet, which is widely exploited all over Europe by call girls and independent escorts. It shows no data regarding trafficking and whether the law has changed activity there. It is at most a puff piece – that the UK government seems keen to use as a model for its own future decisions regarding sex work.

What a lot of people don't know is that the strict laws of the Swedish model are also applied to people living with sex workers. This has long been used as a way to prosecute exploitative potential boyfriends or pimps. But the way the laws are written means that they may include uninvolved family members – and even sex workers' children. There are already cases in which sex workers' children have been charged with pimping because they were living with a sex worker and not paying rent.

Meanwhile, in Canada, laws – and attitudes – are changing. Terri-Jean Bedford, a dominatrix whose brothel the Bondage Bungalow had been subjected to numerous Canadian police raids, court cases, and appeals, finally prevailed in a legal battle that had been going on since the early 1990s.

'It's a great day for Canada. It's like emancipation day for sex trade workers,' Bedford said at a press conference in September 2010. 'You can't imagine how happy I am today because I've been abused by the justice system for a very, very, very long time.'

After two decades defending her right to a livelihood, Bedford's argument found favour with Ontario Superior Court Justice Susan Himel. Himel's judgment ruled that prostitutes' rights to 'life, liberty, and security' under the Canadian Charter of Rights and Freedoms were being violated by aggressive policing.

Like in the UK, prostitution itself is legal in Canada, but many of the activities surrounding it are not. The ruling challenged three laws restricting those activities – keeping a brothel, communicating for the purposes of prostitution, and living off the proceeds of prostitution. In a 132-page ruling, the judge said: 'I find that the danger faced by prostitutes greatly outweighs any harm which may be faced by the public.'[182]

The government side argued that all forms of prostitution are unsafe, and making brothels legal would only attract sex tourists and human traffickers to Canada. But Himel rejected those opinions, stating they were 'issues that are, in my view, incidental to the case …'. She criticised claims made by Melissa Farley for the government's case, saying, 'Some experts made bold assertions without properly outlined bases for their claims and were unwilling to qualify their opinions in the face of new facts provided.' In the summary, Himel confirmed her judgment was supported by two decades of new research.

One of Terri-Jean Bedford's co-complainants, Valerie Scott, said the ruling would allow prostitutes to unionise, protect health and safety, hire protection, and pay income tax. 'We are not aliens. We are ordinary people and now we have rights,' Scott said. 'We can now pick up the phone and call the police and report a bad client.'

Historically, tolerance of prostitution has benefited women who have no other routes to earnings and ownership. As with the failure of the 'War on Drugs' to eliminate either the drug trade or the criminal elements involved in it, the available evidence suggests it is actually criminalisation of prostitution – not prostitution itself – that harms people. Moving sex workers from well-lit situations into dark city outskirts puts them in danger. Decriminalised sex trades can actually drive down sexually transmitted infection rates.

And yet the messages, against not only sex work but also sex workers, suggest otherwise. Reading the arguments of those who want to criminalise prostitution, there seems to be a strong residual streak of judgement and morality at work. While prostitution is thought by many to be a victimless crime, the people who oppose sex work keep claiming all sex workers are victims and that the only solution is criminal punishment.

The style of argument frequently used by opponents of prostitution was summarised by failed Reagan appointee to the US Supreme Court, Robert Bork. In defending the prosecution of victimless crimes, he wrote, 'Knowledge that an activity is taking place is a harm to those who find it profoundly immoral.'[183]

The problem with such an attitude is this: who gets to decide what is and is not profoundly immoral? How many people need to find something profoundly immoral before the police are compelled to prosecute the crime? One thousand? One hundred? One? In such a world the objections of a small yet vocal minority could conceivably hold more power than the opinions of a silent majority.

Considering the broad range of religious and cultural backgrounds represented in Britain today, at least one person somewhere takes offence to just about everything you do in your daily life. It makes no sense to cater to the fear that someone might be morally offended by something they never see and never affects their lives in any real way. A consensus should be reached based on the best available evidence, not on pandering to the sensibilities of the easily offended.

Some criticisms of the sex industry, such as whether there is a danger in commodifying sexuality, are worth talking about. But most of the opposition is blinkered and supports action that does not help the people who are at most risk of exploitation. It is tiresome to listen to the same old moral objections being trotted out, when sex workers are usually more interested in avoiding harassment from police or finding the safest possible way to earn a living.

There is an enormous difference between helping women trapped in cycles of abuse and attacking women whose experiences are off message. Anytime such voices appear – the educated call girl, perhaps, or the self-motivated porn star – they are belittled and marginalised by people who label them as 'rare' or even 'lying'.

But it is not lying if your experience contradicts a well-worn stereotype, and it is not rare to want to be involved in a process that affects your livelihood. Groups like the Asia Pacific Network of Sex Workers (APNSW), or the Desiree Alliance in the US, are made up of sex workers who have much to say about the policies affecting them. They not only include but embrace women whose backgrounds are not privileged and not middle class: in other words, the same people some think need 'saving'.

There are many other groups like the APNSW and Desiree. But they are attacked or ignored by opponents outside of prostitution who prefer selective information bolstering their stereotype of 'broken' and 'vulnerable' women. Opponents who prefer to imply they, not sex workers themselves, know best. Sex workers trying to have a voice in the policy that affects them must feel rather as early suffragettes did, being talked down to by men.

Prohibiting sex work is not a successful behaviour-changing policy. Prohibition in general tends to backfire. We all know how badly alcohol prohibition in the US went. Instead of addressing the underlying social issues that might have been leading to unwelcome levels of alcoholism, it simply gave criminals a far greater hold on the industry than they would have had otherwise. It did little to solve any actual family or societal problems.

The government policy of the last several decades against sex workers has failed. No matter what deterrents are applied, sex work always continues. Even in Sweden, which claims success with its criminalisation strategy. The Swedish government admits sex work advertising has increased on the internet – in other words, the trade has disappeared from public spaces but has not gone away at all. What has happened is that sex workers have gone underground. This makes them more vulnerable, not less, to attack and abuse.

If as a society we are serious about protecting women, then we should rethink the current approach. The only country in the world that has put the safety of women and men in sex work above subjective moral ideals is New Zealand. Its decriminalisation of sex work over ten years ago has been a great success.

In times of financial austerity, throwing more money at unsuccessful policies is against the public interest and out of step with public opinion. Many opinion polls clearly show that people support protecting the safety of sex workers and support decriminalisation. Criminalising consensual sexual activity between adults is wrong and dangerous.

A lot of the debate owes more to ideology than to reality. Much was made of Iceland's decision to close its strip clubs and Sweden's approach to criminalising prostitution. But how does it make sense to attack particular kinds of physical work, when people make money from their bodies in other ways? Surely, by that logic, fashion modelling and ballet dancing ought to be banned as well? There is also an element of these arguments that is strongly gendered. Men's bodies are exploited by war – few people dare endorse putting the Army out of business. There are vulnerable and exploited people in all kinds of work, not just sex work. Surely it makes more sense to attack the conditions that make them vulnerable, not the work they use to try to change their situations.

While Sweden's official figures fail to show that its no-tolerance approach to sex work actually helps anyone, that hasn't stopped some activists from claiming victory. Because in a sense, no matter what happens, it is a victory. A victory for a particular point of view. Not a victory for evidence, not a victory for facts. Certainly not a victory for the people the law actually affects.

The difference between how we imagine prostitutes' lives to be and how they actually are rarely gets airtime. Why? One reason could be because drawing attention to this difference might challenge the agenda of government, NGOs, and certain charities.

The few times when a voice is heard that doesn't fit the stereotype, it is often discounted or ridiculed. Since coming out as a former sex worker, I have been criticised for being too middle class, too well educated, too independent. As if my very existence in sex work was, somehow, unique. But data across the spectrum of sex work shows this not to be true.

It's bizarre to read articles by people who've never met me attempting to dissect this or that bit of my life. Inevitably some lazy commentators 'blame' me for the existence of other call girls, or the idea that smart, driven people might ever consider sex work among their earning options. But, as delightfully flattering as that is, it's not true. Prostitution is called 'the oldest profession' for a reason.

Now, a little story about what the people who purport to care about the women in sex work, who want so badly to 'save' them, actually think.

The online comments following a review in the *Guardian* of the final series of *Secret Diary* were particularly telling. Very quickly the discussion descended not into an assessment of the show's content, but a discussion of me as a person. I know – they need to get over it already. And then there was this one comment in particular:

'The show should end with her dead in a ditch.'

Which had, by the time I saw it, been favourited seventy-four times.

Maybe I was feeling a little oversensitive that day. It wasn't, after all, clear if the commentator thought I should be dead in a ditch, or whether it should just be the person playing me who ends up dead. Whatever. You would be bothered too, if death threats had been delivered to your work after coming out. So I complained to the *Guardian* about the comment, which I felt contravened their website's posting rules. Dozens of other people complained as well. After all, the paper wouldn't have let such comments about a survivor of domestic abuse stand, nor similar jibes about any number of other issues. At the time of writing, the comment had not been removed.

Sex workers are targeted by violent attackers because of an implicit message society as a whole is sending. The comment trivialises murder to the point of implying that someone deserves to die. Simply because they had been a sex worker. That's unspeakably wrong. Not least because it bolsters the conviction of people like Gary Ridgway, who murdered prostitutes because he knew he could get away with it.

I filed a complaint with the Press Complaints Commission, who eventually found in favour of the *Guardian* because, according to them, sex workers are more likely to die while working. So I guess they felt that sort of commentary is a-okay.

Wow. Victim blaming, much? Being a fireman is a dangerous job; any troll commentator snarking that a show about emergency services 'should' end with dead bodies would be beyond the pale. Sex work is not everyone's cup of tea, but it is a job and it is – in Britain – legal. Suck on that, haters. You might think raising an eyebrow when people make dead hooker comments is 'political correctness gone mad'. I happen to know you'd feel differently if it was someone you knew.

It is 100 per cent par for the course since, after all, I had the gall to prove them and their closed-loop, neat-and-tidy judgements wrong. I am a woman. I was a sex worker. I lived in London. I said it was all true and I meant – and mean – Every Single Word.

But enough stories. What matters is fact, and I am as tired as everyone else with endless personal attacks masquerading as reasoned debate on this issue. There is a lot of talk in the political sphere about the need for 'evidence-based policy'. This means rejecting approaches that are moralistic and manipulative. Sex workers – like Michaela Hague – have suffered the tragic consequences of prejudicial social attitudes that lead to bad policy. The prohibition approach has not worked. It will never work. The people who endorse a view in which someone 'should' end up dead are not the ones who should be guiding public opinion on this any longer.

Disliking sex work is not a good enough argument to justify criminalising it. Is there any public interest served by preventing adults from engaging in a consensual transaction for sexual services? No, there is not. Bit like the War on Drugs: making the business profitable only to criminals, awaiting the inevitably grim results, then claiming that it's the drugs themselves, not the laws, that caused it. Few reasonable people believe that line of argument when it comes to drugs. Why does anyone believe it when it comes to sex?

Moral disapproval is a bad basis for policy making. I don't find the idea of taking drugs at all appealing, but I don't assume my own preferences should be the basis for law.

The condescension heaped on people who do sex work is embarrassingly transparent. All this mealy-mouthed 'Oh, but we want to help them, really.' How's that again? By saddling people with criminal records and taking away their children? Do me a favour.

As well as the happy, well-paid prostitutes there are unhappy, poor sex workers in need of support. Society should protect the unwilling and underage from sexual exploitation. We already have laws for that. Maybe they should be more intelligently enforced. But the existence of abuses in some employment sectors does not mean such work should be automatically criminalised. There are people abused and taken advantage of in the food service industry, in construction, in commercial fishing. Nobody suggests making them illegal. Perhaps it's time for us to start seeing that sex work is real work too.

9

MYTH: The people who oppose sex work, pornography, and similar issues are motivated only by what they think is best for society.

'Vice trade a disease time bomb,' yelled one headline.[184] 'Police send STD info to suspects in prostitution sting,' advised another.[185] Even the sports pages were not immune, with 'AIDS and HIV warning to South Africa World Cup fans' featured prominently on the BBC website.[186] The World Cup warnings, in particular, were widespread in the run-up to the football tournament in 2010.

Are the headlines accurate? Are prostitutes spreading sexually transmitted infections? Many believe sex workers play the central role in the transmission of STIs to the general public. But a huge amount of research over the past twenty years counters this belief.

Studies consistently show high rates of condom use in sex work, and low risks of HIV and other STIs for women sex workers.[187] Cohort studies have shown a low incidence of HIV infection in sex workers in Europe (0.2 cases per 100 person years in the United Kingdom).[188] Despite an increase in the rate of STIs in the general population, sex workers have shown a decline in infections.[189] In the Netherlands, where prostitution is legal and workers' health monitored, sex workers have a lower rate of sexually transmitted infections than swingers.[190]

The real vectors are not sex workers, most of whom use condoms, and are tested regularly for infections. In the UK, the population that is really experiencing a surge in STIs is the over-fifties. About

13,000 older men and women were diagnosed with STIs in 2009, double the number diagnosed in 2000.[191] Rather than prostitutes spreading disease, the real vectors seem to be people who assume that their partners are 'safe', or people who were perhaps in committed relationships and marriages the last time public health campaigns about safer sex were saturating the media, but aren't monogamous any more.

Still the headlines continued. 'Prostitutes flock to South Africa ahead of World Cup 2010,' claimed the *Christian Science Monitor*, with similar warnings in the *Washington Post*, *New York Times*, and virtually every English-language international paper. According to reports seeded by social work groups and charities, some 40,000 prostitutes were set to arrive in South Africa – coincidentally, the identical number that had been predicted (but never materialised) for Germany's World Cup in 2006.

Leaked diplomatic cables discuss the sex-trafficking scare around that earlier World Cup. 'Over 20 NGOs throughout Germany have received government funds to conduct dozens of trafficking prevention and awareness campaigns.'[192] The same cable discusses raids on Munich brothels in search of said trafficking victims, noting it couldn't find any. Another cable discusses raids, involving hundreds of police officers, in which seventy-four women were detained. '[P]olice findings demonstrate there has been no substantial increase in [trafficking in persons] and that the oft-repeated figure of 40,000 prostitutes converging on Germany for the FIFA World Cup is a gross exaggeration.' [193]

Despite – or perhaps because of – the hype, German statistics on the total number of confirmed cases of 'human trafficking for the purpose of sexual exploitation' in 2006 are readily available. For the entire country (not only sites around World Cup matches), for the entire year (not only the duration of the World Cup), what is the total? It's five. A monumentally unimpressive 0.0167 per cent of the predicted number that were supposed to occur during the World Cup alone.

This means one of two things: either Germany's law enforcement can't be bothered to do anything about crimes even when warned they are about to occur, or the predictions on sex trafficking produced for the delectation of the media are very far off the mark. Now, I'm no expert on German police, but I know which option I'd put my money on.

So, the numbers don't hold up. And they don't even sound likely, given the size of expected crowds at events like these. Consider the 40,000 meant to have been trafficked for the South Africa World Cup. With the expected number of fans going to the country estimated at 450,000, that just doesn't pass the sniff test. One working girl for every eleven people at the tournament? That's hospitality provision on a level Premier League teams' Christmas parties would envy.

Why were the working girls in South Africa during the World Cup the ones getting all the headlines? And was the hype about a ticking disease time bomb true?

As it happens, the claim about widespread sex tourism was refuted several months later when a UN Population Fund report showed sex workers' activity didn't go up at all.[194]

The very same scare reports about projected trafficking and disease statistics are being recycled in advance of the 2012 London Olympics, with conferences and fundraising events popping up to 'raise awareness'. Early 2011 saw reports of the tens of thousands of women who were 'expected' to be trafficked into Dallas for fans of American football at the Super Bowl. The projected numbers were identical to those supposed to have been trafficked for the World Cup in South Africa, the Ryder Cup in Wales, the 2006 World Cup in Germany, the 2004 Olympics in Athens, and the 2000 Olympics in Sydney. In every one of these examples, the projections have neither been supported by evidence beforehand nor proved to be accurate afterwards. And yet the same stories, the same numbers, and the usual suspects wanting money lurk behind every major sporting event of the last decade and longer.

Which is unsurprising ... because the entire 'World Cup' disease publicity was part of a strategy devised by (among others) Hunt Alternatives Fund to tie international sports headlines to hype about sex work and trafficking.

What is Hunt Alternatives Fund? It is a private foundation started in the 1980s by the daughters of right-wing US oil tycoon HL Hunt. Hunt was a man who believed votes should be distributed to citizens according to their personal wealth. Hunt Alternatives Fund's multi-year campaign attacking sex work was developed with the help of Abt Associates, one of the largest for-profit consulting firms in the world. Abt's other recent activities include accepting a $250-million consulting contract on how to improve health services in Nigeria, and another $121 million to look into the possibility of means-testing people on disability benefits in America.

Abt Associates' input resulted in an action plan that outlined the approach Hunt should take in promoting the criminalisation of sex workers and clients. But rather than relying on hard research, they had a rather more flashy campaign in mind.

Here is a sample from Hunt's own report, *Developing a National Action Plan for Eliminating Sex Trafficking*: '[Hunt Alternatives Fund] should seize large marketing opportunities, such as the upcoming World Cup matches in South Africa, to create controversy on a world level and use it to draw attention to prostitution.'[195] As a PR stunt, it worked. Speculative reports about tourism and prostitution were far more widely reported than the UN's evidence-based contradiction of these claims.

In the Hunt document these recommendations come under the heading of 'Demand Reduction as an Effective Public Health Inter-vention', or in other words, push the myth that sex workers are re-sponsible for STIs. But spreading rumours about disease is only one plan. Other sections cover 'Emphasizing Sexual Exploitation of Children Versus Adults' – so that's keeping the focus on child abuse, regardless of the actual issues – and 'Establish a National Center Devoted to Combating Demand', since these recommen-dations would presumably do better with a 'centre' to give them legitimacy.

The Hunt/Abt strategy values political lobbying far above sound evidence. 'With severe time and resources constraints, lawmakers should not be asked to do the groundwork and raise support. Instead, a coalition and political advocates should present them with the issue, easily packaged and understood.' Also, never underestimate the power of celebrity: 'Several celebrities are already involved or interested in combating demand, such as Ashley Judd, Ashton Kutcher, and Demi Moore.'

The Hunt guidelines note that finding evidence to support their viewpoint might be difficult. 'The point is that the "gold standard" usually is costly, and is not always feasible to pursue,' according to the document. 'The challenge in establishing standards of evidence is in determining the level or type of evidence required to convince [those organisations] sponsoring the programs.' Or, in other words, find the lowest acceptable level of evidence, and pursue only that. And, if in doubt, avoid conducting studies at all: 'No new information is necessarily required, so there is no need to wait for new research to unfold.'

It's possible that many of the people who oppose sex for money have the best possible, if misguided, intentions. Hunt Alternatives Fund, for instance, declares that its main aim is to 'advance inclusive approaches to social change'.

In case there was any doubt about how Hunt Alternatives Fund feels about the people in sex work, and whether this 'inclusive change' extends to them, the guidelines speak for themselves. When discussing the words that should be used to describe people having sex for money, the document recommends sticking to 'prostituted person, sexually exploited, sex slaves'.

In Hunt's view, there is no way to distinguish between willing and unwilling sex workers, so why bother trying? 'When addressing demand that drives sexual slavery, it is not possible to separate the buyers of compelled sex from those whose participation is not due to force, fraud, or coercion.' This assumes that no participants in sex work have any agency. That solely by the act of having sex for money, one is rendered incapable of self-determination. That's a ludicrous assumption, with nothing to support it.

So when the document says, 'If the National Campaign is to be comprehensive, it will require numerous partners from diverse backgrounds engaging in many different collective activities.' That presumably excludes all people who have a positive experience of sex work.

The people who oppose prostitution on principle not only produce suspect research, but feel that rhetoric better suits their campaign than facts. Looking over the list of contributors to Hunt Alternatives Fund, one sees many familiar names: *Guardian* writer Julie Bindel, Gail Dines, Melissa Farley. Conspicuously absent is any input from women in sex work themselves. Imagine if a similar document outlining how to tackle the international problem of sexism was signed only by men? There'd be an uproar.

Also absent are any of the numerous academics who do not demonise sex work as a precondition of their research. No independent academics have been called to give evidence to any of the recent government committees examining prostitution.

And the pay for putting one's name to this document is, apparently, not bad either. On Twitter I asked Julie Bindel if she found her alliance with Hunt to be a lucrative one – 'Absolutely lucrative as fuck!' was the reply.[196] Ironic, isn't it, for such a vocal opponent of sex work to be so pleased to be in it for the money?

Hunt Alternatives and Abt Associates are not the only groups using this kind of approach. The Schapiro Group, a market research firm in the US, regularly produces press releases with an anti-sex-work bias. And their publications have been used to influence US policy on sex workers and advertising.

In September 2010, the popular website Craigslist was forced to remove its adult advertising section after explosive testimony to the US Congress. Deborah Richardson of the Women's Funding Network, which commissioned Schapiro to conduct the study, told legislators that juvenile prostitution is exploding at an astronomical rate. And she laid the blame at the door of websites like Craigslist.

'An independent tracking study released today by the Women's Funding Network shows that over the past six months, the number of underage girls trafficked online has risen exponentially in three diverse states,' Richardson claimed. 'Michigan: a 39.2 per cent increase; New York: a 20.7 per cent increase; and Minnesota: a staggering 64.7 per cent increase.' National papers like *USA Today*, the Houston *Chronicle*, the Miami *Herald*, and the Detroit *Free Press* all repeated the dire warnings as gospel.

What is the Schapiro Group? Perhaps it's easiest to explain that the Schapiro Group's other main activity is conducting 'push polls' for conservative candidates in the US. Push polling means cold-calling voters supposedly to assess their political leanings in an upcoming election, with the real agenda of 'pushing' a particular point of view.

Push polling is a strange business. It's also one I've experienced first hand. As a poor student, I briefly worked in an establishment that used such tactics, and quit as soon as humanly possible. That call centre used every trick in the book, from misrepresenting ourselves, to lying about our location, to asking loaded questions. One I recall in particular was, 'Would you be more, or less inclined to vote for the Democrat candidate if you knew he was involved in money laundering?' Of course, the man in question had never been accused of such a thing. But the question was cleverly written to avoid a legal challenge, and also to invoke a particular response. That was the year of the surprise success of Republican House leader Newt Gingrich and his conservative 'Contract With America'. I was sickened to think my job had contributed to that in any way.

Considering the culture of push polling, it's no surprise that Schapiro's results look frightening, until you critically assess the details. As with much push polling, definitions are stretched, and assumptions are relied upon. One study defined 'adolescents' as anyone up to the age of twenty-two. Another focused on 'child sexual exploitation' of people one and two years over the age of consent.[197]

Another study estimates the number of teenagers in escorting, but look carefully – they don't have any actual data on age. So, where do their numbers come from? Guesses of age, based on photos in escort ads! Even they admit this method is laughably unreliable. 'The problem is, there is no scientifically reliable previous experience on which to base the probability that a girl selling sex who looks quite young is, indeed, under eighteen years.' Doesn't stop them from writing an entire report in which they do exactly that, mind.

While the information given to legislators focused on child exploitation, there was no evidence that children were being exploited on Craigslist. Rather, the issue appears to have been used as a smokescreen to obtain the *real* desired result: eliminating consensual adult sex work. And it's done by fudging the details and hiding behind the smokescreen of protecting children.

No one supports child sexual exploitation, but stretching the term to include people who are legally adults is manipulative and disingenuous. It also deflects attention from the real abusers of actual children.

Shutting down websites and spreading misinformation is undoubtedly far easier than doing the real work of stopping exploitation. Closing down adult ads on sites like Craigslist gets attention. Hollywood stars getting their mates to front flashy 'awareness' campaigns gets attention. High-profile raids, high-drama invented statistics, and Congressional hearings get attention. The real victims don't.

But as far as Hunt Alternatives, Abt Associates, and the Schapiro Group are concerned, thin research is good enough for them.

'There is no "other side" of the argument,' claims the Hunt document. In spite of evidence that 60 per cent of British people think prostitution should be the choice of the person doing it, not the government.[198] 'They have no credible supporters', claims Hunt. Who's calling who not credible again? When Hunt comes out of its own reports looking like just one more group promoting minimal research standards and celebrity endorsement over intellectually honest evidence.

Unfortunately for Hunt Alternatives Fund, the celebrity train does not always pull into the station as smoothly as planned. Some people who don't need the money seem to be in it for the credibility boost.

Hollywood stars Demi Moore and Ashton Kutcher unveiled their DNA Foundation charity in 2010. The centrepiece was a barrage of viral adverts, fronted by some of the famous couple's friends. Justin Timberlake, Ed Norton, and Sean Penn all lent their star power to the 'Real Men Don't Buy Girls' campaign.

On its face, the aim of the DNA foundation is to support efforts against forced sex trafficking. However, its remit also affects consensual sex workers. They don't seem to mind. On Quora.com, Kutcher contributed an answer to the question 'Why is it so common to include voluntary prostitution in the category of sex trafficking?' Not only did his answer reference some of the most commonly repeated myths about sex work, one of his supporters even used me as an example![199]

If there's one thing I'm definitely opposed to, it's being used against my will by people who attack the sex industry. Just being mentioned in that discussion made me feel more in need of a delousing than any experience as a call girl ever did.

Anyway, the *Village Voice* published an article refuting some of Kutcher's more flimsy claims under the heading 'Real Men Get Their Facts Straight'.[200] Kutcher retaliated by launching a tirade against the *Voice*, pressuring advertisers to pull their money because of the Backpage.com sex worker listings, which he claimed had been used for underage trafficking (the one case that was threatened against the *Voice* was thrown out of court).[201]

The usual disclaimer … I am (as indeed all of Kutcher's critics are) opposed to forced trafficking in any form, including child sex trafficking. But we must not let emotion exclusively carry the day; it achieves nothing. The *Voice* hits the nail on the head with this summary of DNA's work in their original article: 'An emotional reaction, based on good intentions, but grounded in bogus information.'

The problem of bogus information is this – campaigns such as Kutcher's conflate all sex work with child sex trafficking. Approaches that do so not only encourage criminalisation legislation that harms consenting adults, but also obscures the real victims. How? By using vastly inflated numbers for one kind of trafficking, and pretty much ignoring everything else. Actual children being actually trafficked for actual sex are rarely, if ever, found by the kind of scattershot brothel raids and streetwalker crackdowns so many seem to consider 'successes' in the anti-trafficking effort.

Kutcher, while earnest, is propagating harmful myths. The raids on brothels are not successful in stopping trafficking. They are vast wastes of time, money, and manpower. And many groups receiving funding meant to help victims of trafficking seem instead to be picking and choosing who is worthy of their largesse.

There is undoubtedly work to be done eliminating forced trafficking of men and women for *any* kind of labour. But the approach required almost certainly isn't the one anti-traffickers think will work. Making sex work illegal has never been shown to eliminate or even lessen forced sex trafficking.

Kutcher's response to the *Voice* inspired loads of his millions of followers to join in Tweeting criticism to advertisers. So far, so 'concerned'. And then, when the *Voice* didn't respond directly to him, he Tweeted:

@aplusk
ashton kutcher

No Response @villagevoice **? Oh I forgot U work business hrs. Maybe that's Y you sell girls on ur platform. they tend 2work the night shift**

Like a lot of people, Ashton Kutcher seems to have some pretty confused ideas about sex work. To be in a position of wanting to help people, yet still falling back on uninformed stereotypes when talking about them, is inexcusable. Someone who writes on his blog, 'I've spent the last two years meeting with every expert on the issue of Human Trafficking that I can find, reading countless books, meeting with victims and former traffickers,' should maybe know better.[202] Perhaps Ashton could have made time for a little bit of victim sensitivity training in there somewhere?

I know a little about what it's like to be asked to comment on issues you don't necessarily have expertise in. Sometimes, journalists and television shows approach people like me to provide commentary rather than, say, academics in the relevant fields. It's unfortunate but it's a fact of media life. And I do try, by following academic discussions and talking with friends who are professionals in, say, sex education or the porn industry, to at least not come off as too much of an ignorant tit.

I would shudder in horror, though, to ever be described (as Moore and Kutcher have by CNN) as a 'leading player' in the debate around such serious issues. But maybe in a weird way Kutcher is, with significant numbers of his followers joining in his Twitter tirade, and the man himself being promoted as somehow more of an expert on sex work than people who have devoted entire working or academic lives to the field.

Not bad for a guy whose credentials, according to his Twitter profile, are: 'I make stuff up.'

The well-meaning Twitter fans following Kutcher's lead probably don't realise they might be being taken for a ride on the facts front. It can be very hard to sort the real from the fake when people keep repeating made-up stuff about sex work as true.

Issues such as trafficking are hot topics for people who claim their main motivation is to help those involved. Help is a great thing. There are loads of people who could all use a little help, in all professions and walks of life.

On one hand, many of the people concerned about the welfare of sex workers are no doubt motivated by a genuine desire to help others. Particularly those they think of as unable to defend themselves. But the flipside of this is that charities need money to survive. As other charities have discovered in the past, sometimes the desire to have a high profile and keep the wheels greased overtakes the benefit to the people you are trying to help.

High-profile media reports have shown how the money given from individuals' pockets may not end up where they expect. The people who might be considered most in need are, often, at the bottom of a very long list.

For instance, how many people supporting Bono's high-profile charity efforts were shocked to read, in the *New York Post*, that less than $500,000 of the $15 million raised by his non-profit organisation, the ONE Campaign, ended up in the hands of the individuals that organisation is established to help. The rest, according to the paper, was spent on other things including black tie galas, salaries and expenses, and pricey incentives and gifts to inspire donors. For every $30 given, it was reported that only $1 went where many original donors might have hoped it would.

A spokesman for the charity, Oliver Buston, came out to defend ONE, saying the money is used for raising awareness. 'We don't provide programmes on the ground. We're an advocacy and campaigning organisation,' said Buston. The honourable intentions of the ONE Campaign are not in doubt but whether many donors were fully aware of this focus at the time they gave is open to debate.

Charity funding is something of a minefield. Charities vary widely in how their money gets distributed and in how much makes it to the purported beneficiary. While high-drama concerns such as abuse and trafficking can pluck at the heart- (and purse-) strings, it's interesting to examine where exactly the money comes from, and where it's ending up.

There is no reason to think Constellation Makers produce misleading statistics with the sole intent of abusing the public's trust. If anything, their intentions are probably well meaning on some level. Still, there is a motivation that goes beyond altruism: money. Researchers can study a crisis; advocacy groups claiming to address it can get grants and support; stories related to sex and sex work sell papers.

While many people are motivated by their beliefs or by a sense that they need to be seen to be doing something, it is also true that without money, it's pretty hard to get anything done. You can't further an agenda without something greasing the wheels, and it's always worth following the money.

Charities and other groups that purport to 'attack' the problem of sex work and 'save' the victims of trafficking are little different. For all the good work they purport to do, there is also a network of high-profile campaigns, conferences, and media-friendly PR that eats up rather a lot of the money donated – including money given by the government.

How some manage to profit from the prostitution and trafficking panics is interesting. A total of £100,000 was allocated by the government to the Poppy Project to support victims identified by Pentameter Two – on top of the over £2 million it already received in funding and the £5.8 million overall given to its parent project, Eaves.[203, 204] At the time of the operation, their facilities in London included thirty-five beds. Thirty-five seems rather a low number if they were expecting the police to find thousands of trafficked women.

The credibility gap when it comes to human sex trafficking doesn't stop at the numbers of supposed victims. The amount of money being thrown at the issue, and what it's used for, are also suspect. In the past decade over forty human trafficking task forces have been established in the US, using money allocated by the federal government. However, none of them were required to collect any data, nor even prove the existence of a local trafficking problem before securing grants. It was January 2008 before these task forces were required to report any activity to the US Bureau of Justice Statistics.[205]

The task forces also had very few restrictions on how their funds could be used. For instance, it would be acceptable for a task force to, say, purchase 'designated vehicles' and fund 'deputy' positions even without a single reported victim of trafficking in the community.

In 2011, Iowa senator Chuck Grassley called for action after audits showed recipients of human trafficking grants reporting questionable costs. The audits showed that of the $8.24 million total the Department of Justice awarded to six grant recipients, there was $2.72 million in unsupported, unallowable, or questioned costs. 'These select individual audits signal to me that there is a bigger problem', said Grassley during a Senate Judiciary Committee hearing. 'Before we reauthorise another dollar, we need strong oversight language included in legislation – to ensure that failing grantees will not be rewarded with additional taxpayer dollars.'

One audit discovered that the Heartland Alliance for Human Needs in Chicago, which was awarded $2 million, spent $902,122 on salaries and $174,479 for 'fringe benefits' – amounts for which they did not have appropriate authorisation. An audit carried out in 2008 found that although the Office of Justice Programs' human grant recipients have 'built significant capacities to serve victims', the programmes have not 'identified and served significant numbers of victims'.[206]

In February 2011, Denise Marshall, chief executive of Eaves Housing for Women and the Poppy Project (which funds Lilith R&D, of the questionable lap-dancing statistics), handed back an OBE she received in 2007. Marshall said it was in protest at the funding cuts her organisation was experiencing under the coalition government. 'We will see situations where women are in danger as a result of the cuts', said Marshall in a newspaper interview. 'We have always worked on a shoestring, but now that shoestring has been cut.'[207]

The shoestring Marshall refers to included £1.95 million of

government funding in 2010. And while coverage of Marshall returning her gong makes it sound as if all money is being cut, the reality is that government funding makes up only some of Eaves' funding. In 2010 their income, according to the Charities Commission website, was about £5.4 million.[208] They've launched a new fundraising drive to recover some of the funds lost from the government grants, as well.

In 2011, it was announced that the government contract for providing services to trafficked individuals had gone from Eaves' Poppy Project to the Salvation Army. There are concerns about what the change will mean, as the Salvation Army's philosophy is more faith-orientated than most people would be comfortable with. But as Nelson Jones wrote for Heresy Corner in April 2011, 'Eaves might not disturb the peace and quiet of your local high street by banging tambourines, but their evangelical zeal is, if anything, even greater than the Sally Army's.'[209]

This observation was also made in 2009, when Belinda Brooks-Gordon, writing for the *Guardian*, commented on the relationship of Eaves with the Labour government and their stated aim to 'be recognised as one of the leading agencies on violence against women issues'. As Brooks-Gordon wrote, 'one fears this implies corporate domination over the interests of, rather than provision of service to, women.'[210]

We must consider that the Salvation Army could provide services for men and for women, since after all, trafficking is not only the sex trafficking of women. And that Eaves' facilities for trafficking victims – which contained fewer than fifty beds – were reportedly accessible only to people who contributed to police investigations. Plenty of folks have reservations about such criteria for accessing services, with good reason.

Everyone wants to see trafficking investigated correctly and intelligently, but holding out services on condition of police co-operation? That would be a little like telling rape victims that only the ones who go to court deserve counselling. Or telling domestic abuse victims they can only go to shelters if they go to the police first. Not a great idea in so, so many ways.

Some have questioned their policy of encouraging police investigation. As Laurie Penny wrote in 2008, 'Feminists and sex workers alike have been appalled at the insistence by members of the Project that prostitutes agree to give up sex work forever and to turn in their traffickers – sometimes a very dangerous step for them to take – before they receive any help whatsoever.' This is 'highly conditional help', to use Penny's words. [211]

Other observations questioned the cost-effectiveness of such a system against the assets that could be seized and the number of people helped. In 2009, Liberal Conspiracy hit out about the money said to be involved: '£1.8 million per year in prosecution costs and £2.1-£3.4 million for a national referral system and specialist victim support services against £1.2 million a year recouped from projected seizures of traffickers' assets ... all of which is based on this new system dealing with 500 trafficked adults and 360 trafficked children a year. A figure that appears, like the estimated unit cost of providing these support services, to have been derived exclusively from information provided by the Poppy Project.' [212]

There are many excellent charities for women's services run by committed staff and volunteers – and fantastic people within every organisation. And there are others whose reliance on media attention and government grants has perhaps damaged their effectiveness.

The bun fight currently going on over funding to help trafficking victims is one example, pitting London-centric feminists from Eaves against evangelical Big Society projects from the Salvation Army.

When the main recipient of anti-trafficking funding is a self-professed feminist organisation that mainly offers its services to women in London, then something has gone wrong, and there are people who will suffer as a result. When the only competitor for the government grants to fund such work is an evangelical outfit ... well, that is a choice I am glad I don't have to make.

Charities aside – and, let it be said, there are many worthy and honest ones – there are also the academics, researchers, and writers who earn their living not through hands-on effort, but by writing papers. Papers that allow them to win grants. Grants so that they can write more papers.

This, as a former cancer research academic, is a world I know well. We can't all save lives. But we do all have to earn a crust. Still, sometimes the ratio of money available to size of the problem seems far out of whack. You do start to wonder how much of what is said and written is born from genuine concern, and how much is just chasing another year's salary.

Is there enough money in these grants to even bother making this criticism? Well, thanks to a little tool that compares the money from funding grants over time, we can make a rough guess of what they are worth. The website Fundingtrends.org, a US-based site, shows trends in research grants funded since 1991. The site processes project-funding data from the US National Institutes of Health (NIH), European Commission (EC), Canadian and Australian research councils, and many others. It also includes keywords from MEDLINE article abstracts, forming an overview of what kinds of research are being funded, and what the amounts involved are.

The site demonstrates that funding for studying trafficking is a growth area. From almost nothing in 1991, it was funded worldwide by 2010 to the tune of over $1 billion. This is a total greater than the amount of grant money awarded to study lung cancer, which of course is also devastating, and affects far more people.[213] And spending on trafficking since 2000 has dwarfed the grant awards on such important international health concerns as malnutrition, malaria, or tuberculosis – conditions that kill millions of people worldwide every year, and affect hundreds of millions more. Funding for trafficking research is not only greater than each of these, it's greater than all of the funding for these health crises *combined*.[214]

This trend has happened at the same time mentions of trafficking started to become interesting to the media. According to a recent article, news database searches showed there were only three references to 'human trafficking' or 'trafficking in humans' before 2000. It was mentioned 9 times in 2000 and 41 times in

2001. Use of these terms in the news reached 100 mentions for the first time in 2005. In 2010, there were more than 500 references.[215]

While trafficking is a serious concern, there is a lot to be said for the benefits of even modest funding saving far more people when it comes to issues like controlling TB, or attacking malnutrition. They are not sexy but they are just as, if not more, important. In countries where trafficking is the most rife, health concerns like these are often far more acutely serious in day-to-day life. It's a bit like chucking loads of money at education, only to learn no one's too bothered about the fact the school itself is burning down.

Another way in which opposing sex work brings financial benefit is through the Proceeds of Crime Act 2002. Police know, for instance, that if a brothel owner is prosecuted, since running a brothel is illegal, any money and property retrieved from the 'crime scene' becomes theirs. When police resources are limited, does the temptation of profit possibly influence victimless crimes being prosecuted more vigorously than they otherwise would? Hard to know for sure. It's to no one's surprise that the pre-Olympic crackdown on brothels is coinciding with the recent cuts in police funding.

Hanna Morris, who ran a brothel, lost her 'abuse of process' case against the police. She rang 999 when masked and armed gunmen threatened her business ... only to find herself arrested, and the violent criminals never pursued or apprehended.[216] It's impossible to know for certain, but one can imagine plenty of situations in which police – with restricted time and money – must make choices: unknown violent criminals who may be difficult and expensive to catch, or women technically breaking the law standing right in front of you, with cash assets?

The outcome of the Morris case certainly sends a message, but I'm not convinced it's the message of 'protecting women' that some people prefer to promote.

It's an approach that shows lack of compassion for people in real trouble, and puts the agenda of the rescuer above what's best for the victim.

*

There are plenty of examples of policies that are neither wanted nor needed by the general public being implemented. So, why do they exist?

Writing off issues like the hype around child sexualisation, or sex trafficking, as purely motivated by emotion would be an easy thing to do. But it's not quite accurate, even if the data is misleading and at times entirely made up. These ideas actually take hold by following a set of steps that appears very logical to the parties involved. That process includes, crucially, the public.

The first connection between Agenda Setters and policy making is, of course, the politicians. Agenda Setters know that appealing directly to policy makers enables them to gain sizeable grants or contracts for relatively small investments. Politicians reasonably believe they have more to gain than to lose by supporting these kinds of agendas. They are not so much public servants as self-interested agents. Policies may be tied to campaign contributions, or other forms of implied support, such as lobbying positions or chairmanships after leaving public office. The cost of supporting these projects is low, since politicians are spending the public's money. They also know that few voters are strictly one-issue voters.

The evidence they demand before changing laws, such as through consultations, is rather shoddy only because the outcome is usually already decided bar a few details. Why invest more in research, when everyone involved has already decided what will happen?

On the local scale, it's hard for Agenda Setters to exercise their influence in the same way as they do on the national scale. Partly this is because local interactions have more of an element of getting along, of maintaining community cohesion. These are not always compatible with the way politics works on the macro level. Paying off a school's headteacher in order to implement local internet censorship, for instance, wouldn't go down awfully well, even if people did agree with the result of the policy.

This is where the Constellation Makers and Evangelisers are vital to the process of gaining consent for an agenda, or at least, the appearance of consent.

Constellation Makers provide the vital content that is needed to ensure that if people are concerned about this issue at all, their opinions will be the 'right' ones. Ask yourself, for instance, why the parents consulted for sexualisation research are only asked about sexualisation and never whether it's a big concern to them. That way, the outcome can be presented in a sterile context with no relationship to family life.

The data appear to be asking whether parents think the internet or lads' mags are more dangerous for children. What it doesn't ask is whether either of those rate highly on a parental list of concerns about dangers to their children overall. Realistically, parents are unlikely to feel the content of advertising is the most pressing problem on their plates. The results of the consultations, however, are presented in such a way as to make it look like it's all they think about.

This is where Evangelisers enter the fray. By supplying the media with a large number of articles discussing sex education and sexualisation as the most pressing concern parents have to face, the scene is set for people to start prioritising these issues above, say, the quality of teaching or the success of curricula at the local schools. Newspapers, television news, even the internet are all subject to a certain bandwidth: whether the number of column inches, the amount of time on air, or simply the amount of time spent online.

Pushing out competing information is an effective way of manufacturing consent on these issues. With many members of the public having never considered the issues in depth at all – they're understandably busy – the first thing they see is already prepped and primed to invoke the strongest possible reaction. And those who see the stories but suspect the data in them is somehow not entirely kosher have little access to the resources that might confirm their suspicions.

Finally, the public have a stake in this as well: the perceived time and energy it takes to overcome what is, in isolation, a relatively small slight far outweighs the perceived benefits of whatever government is currently in power. People whose livelihoods are insecure tend to focus energy on improving their specific situations; people whose livelihoods are secure are reluctant to rock the boat. Collective action against these measures is made very difficult. To be ignorant of the minute detail of policies is a rational decision for members of the public. The voices of vocal minorities with the most to gain are prioritised over those of the indifferent majority.

10

CONCLUSION:

While many of the debates in this book have little in common apart from the 'sex' bit, they tend to get lumped together in the eyes of the public, government, and media as something that is affecting society more than before. And it is very often implied that it needs attention *now*. Conflating porn use, sex work, trafficking, and other issues allows Agenda Setters to push a view of the world in which virtually every human interaction is sexually charged – and potentially dangerous.

But the grand plans of Agenda Setters and the ideologically driven Constellation Makers would be nowhere without the helping hand of those happy to spread the word. We want answers. We like answers. Media strive to give us answers, even if they're not entirely correct. The complex and indefinable truth rarely, if ever, gets a look-in.

How things are reported can have an outsize influence on what people believe about these issues, and how prominent they are seen to be. In the quest to fill pages and cut costs, few are able to devote the time to accurately checking stories as they should, and press releases are frequently taken at face value. There is a tendency to re-report information even long after it has been discredited. Making sure every side is represented often results in emotive arguments being given the same weight as factual material. Also, some journalists summarise without even checking their sources.

This completes the circle: Agenda Setters defined the problem, Constellation Makers set the boundaries of its existence, and Evangelisers spread the word. The concerned public rises up in what appears to be a grassroots fashion to put pressure on Agenda Setters to solve this terrible – and previously completely unknown – problem.

As a science student, I was taught early the value of original sources. A science education is a little like the history of science: you spend your school and university years working through well-known experiments, amassing first-hand knowledge, and learning how to read and interpret research findings. Then, if you stick with it, you get to go on and do your own research someday.

It's not only science where this happens. Disciplines like history, for example, place high value on the original source. But almost everything you read in the news media is a summary or an interpretation. How good are those summaries and interpretations? Being able to read and interpret information for yourself is important – vitally so. Because there's not enough time in the day for each and every one of us to do that for everything we're interested in. Hence, the news media has a place of importance as a translator of news and ideas to the public.

Yet our sources of information are often themselves recycling misinterpreted bits and parts from half-remembered and half-understood things. A newspaper covers a politician's letter, which then becomes a source that enters the parliamentary discussion, the transcript of which itself becomes evidence for another newspaper article. The debacle over misestimated trafficking numbers is an excellent example of this. The cycle is seemingly endless, and how real data get into the loop is anyone's guess.

In day-to-day life, it might not even be all that important. But when the discussion affects how serious crimes like trafficking are viewed, or is used to enact policies that victimise women, well … it might be worth returning to the source now and then.

Along with the news media, feminism also has a charge to answer here. By focusing on problems of sex and sexuality to the exclusion of social justice, the aims of feminism have gone far from where they began. And by narrowing that focus even more exclusively to problems in the West or of privileged women, there is a danger of ignoring legitimately worrying trends simply because the majority of self-professed feminists do not relate to them.

Over and again I was surprised to find that the closer I looked at each of these issues, it often seemed to be right-wing religious Agenda Setters and left-wing ideological feminists working to further much the same ends. And I had to wonder why.

One of the most interesting books I have ever read is *The Hand-maid's Tale* by Margaret Atwood. It's a novel about a dystopian future America (called Gilead) in which women are categorised by their value as reproductive objects. The story focuses on the Wives of powerful men, the men's concubines (their Handmaids), and the Jezebels and Unwomen who cannot be integrated into this new, fundamentalist society.

One thing the book touches on is the coalition of far-right and far-left ideals that results in the oppression of women in Gilead. People in the middle, who had no particular investment or opinion either way, got caught in the resulting military dictatorship. They probably approved of some of the early stages without looking into the motives of the people behind them, and implicitly endorsed a future they probably didn't want to live in.

Reproduction in Gilead is regulated by the idea that sex is inherently degrading to women. The book references a past (our present) in which feminists teamed up with conservatives in campaigns against pornography. The consequences of this alliance, however, only empowered feminism's worst enemies. Descriptions of the narrator's feminist mother burning books – then being sent to labour camps as an Unwoman – show feminism allying itself with the religious right, then being discarded by those 'allies'.

When I read this as a teenager it was powerful food for thought. Also, it was kind of nice to read a sci-fi book told exclusively from a woman's perspective, by an authentic female voice. A lot of sci-fi has too much allegory about it for my taste, and the women all end up as traitors or queens. It was refreshing to read a book that had a point to make, but made it with the voice of someone who did not know what the 'right' or 'correct' thing was, nor had a particular moral agenda. Offred, the narrator, is in many ways only a vessel. Anyway.

Silly as it seems, the book has greatly influenced how I interpret, well, loads of stuff. In particular the types of people making the arguments against adult entertainment, against sex work. The right can't decide if you need to be in prison or saved; the left, whether you need to be in a shelter or an 'exiting' programme. There are few accepted stories for sex workers other than Criminal or Victim. There are so many more nuances to issues beyond 'porn bad, children good'.

The more closely you look at the key players behind some of the stories popping up, the more you notice some odd pairings. A group working closely with the anti-gay, anti-abortion US lobbying group using a female MP as the mouthpiece of their opinions on the internet and porn. The well-known UK feminists lending their names to international groups with unknown agendas. Celebrities lending star power to issues they don't understand all that well.

Consider, for instance, a column in the left-leaning *Guardian* of August 2011. Titled 'Should Feminists Back Michele Bachmann?' it suggests with an apparently straight face that support of US presidential candidate Bachmann – an anti-abortion 'surrendered wife' who opposes government provision of healthcare and believes homosexuality can be 'cured' – is a good idea. Why? For the sole reason that she is a woman. To me that's a silly conclusion, sacrificing intellectual honesty on the altar of ideological purity. Being dedicated to tokenism at the highest levels of achievement has clearly altered any sensible view of what the presidency of such a woman would actually mean for the kinds of people the *Guardian* claims to support. But what is clear is that rationalising such potentially undermining choices is far from rare in modern feminism.

And yet there are interesting parallels between the fundamentalist, right-wing US Tea Party types, and the more radical versions of feminism making mainstream headway. That is, in both cases, these are groups that perceive themselves as outsiders. In doing so, they paint themselves as marginalised rebels shaking up a system they feel holds them back (when in fact it nurtures them). Everyone else is held to account, but if you're a victim, seemingly anything goes. And that appears to include all kinds of unholy alliances.

There's a saying where I come from: you got to dance with the one who brung you. I wonder, when everyone gets to the end of their

particular activities, or earn money from their looks. For me, there is more than a little aftertaste of schoolyard gossip in these books. Who's a real feminist, who's just a jumped-up slag?

The slut-shaming attitude is implied in Levy's conclusions, when she says of women who have 'their vaginas waxed … their breasts enlarged': 'I wish them many blissful and lubricious loops around the pole.'

As I read it, she's fine with the idea that there are *some* women who get Brazilians – just as long as they are fine with the idea that she will judge them for that. Rather than imagining pole dancing can co-exist with a brain – or recognising that the privilege of feminism is being permitted to do and think whatever one wishes to do and think – Levy appears to write off the *some* women making superficial and aesthetic choices different from hers. Prim and proper, ladies, that's the way to be! Same as it ever was.

In *Female Chauvinist Pigs*, Levy begins by collecting many anecdotes. She visits the set of *Girls Gone Wild* in Miami. She watches *Charlie's Angels*. She has seen *Nuts* and *FHM* on the shelves; she talked with an editor of the US television series *The Man Show*. She compares these experiences to her own recollections of life at a private New England college in the 1990s, where someone could have been 'pretty much' expelled for using the word 'girl' instead of 'woman'. She saw someone walking down the street wearing a Playboy Bunny shirt, and made her conclusions: sexualisation is more rife than ever and the effects are damaging.

To my eyes, she tells a lot of stories, but does not offer much new in the way of either analysis or substance. Important research is hinted at, but the data never broken down comprehensively. What the reader gets instead are impressions, feelings … anecdotes. And Levy is not the only one who appears to be using this approach.

Natasha Walter, in *Living Dolls* as I read it, seems to spend most of her time preoccupied with the contents of other people's diaries and bemoaning New Labour. Jessica Valenti's *Full Frontal Feminism* is definitely about feminism, but the title seems to promise something new – something that, for me, the book doesn't deliver. And Kat Banyard, in *The Equality Illusion*, opens each chapter with what one review called 'a quasi fictional description of a girl or woman touched by each of the issues under discussion'.[217] Quasi fictional? How about some facts? I rather like Kat as a person and respect her focus; I expected better from her.

Possibly the single most grating thing about the recent spate of women-in-crisis books? The covers. While it's true that few authors have complete control over their covers, these books tend to have pink, glittery covers, predictably emblazoned with a woman's silhouette like cheap pulp fiction. (The conspicuous exception being Banyard's *The Equality Illusion*.) What message do covers like these seem to send? A depressingly reductive one. A message of 'We're going to win you over to our way of thinking, by using exactly the same tactics we criticise other people for.'

In Broadsheet, the 'women's blog' of the popular online news source Salon, I see the contempt as particularly above board. 'There's a new and efficient way to become a published author: sleep with a famous male celebrity!' spits one piece of May 2010 in which a million-dollar publishing deal for one of Tiger Woods' mistresses is derided ... along-side recent books about Norman Mailer by Norris Church Mailer and Carole Mallory, both notable writers in their own right.[218] The implicit message? Write about a famous man and you've sold us out, sister.

One can only assume what a writer that spiteful would make of talented historian Lady Antonia Fraser, who has written about her adulterous relationship with Harold Pinter, or indeed the affairs and polyamory informing much of Simone de Beauvoir's writing. And the Bloomsbury Group? Probably right out.

There's a kind of schizophrenia in modern feminism. On the one hand, we're told that anyone who believes women and men should have equal rights under the law is a feminist, 'whether they know it or not'. On the other, we're told that one or another group is made up of 'gender traitors'. It's hard to reconcile the fact that I believe in equal rights regardless of sex, with the very loud voices calling people like me enemies of feminism.

Capital-F Feminism is a brand few people identify with, while small-f feminism is still an ideal most people support. Unfortunately, that distinction is sometimes lost on the more vocal elements within feminism. It leads to an atmosphere that pushes away more potential allies than it draws in.

Because of this, feminism has real problems with women who don't buy its entire ideology wholesale. Its desire to embrace all women is undermined by its compulsion to demonise a large percentage of them. It marches in the streets for the right to 'reclaim' the word slut in the popular Slutwalks. It also marches in the streets for the right to belittle and ridicule Playboy Bunnies outside a club in London.

In case the irony here isn't clear, the Bunnies are being judged by feminist protesters 1) on account of their sexy appearance and 2) on account of their appearance alone. The thing they are guilty of is doing a legal job for pay which, while not rocket science, is at least a good use of some people's inborn talents. In other words, there is a lot of cheek in decrying people who use 'slut shaming' to belittle women whilst doing the exact same thing yourself. The right to demonstrate is important, but increasingly these demonstrations take the tone of attack and use the language of abuse.

And, of course, there's the usual lambasting from people who think that people like me or like the Playboy Bunnies are not proper women. Thus it's entirely reasonable, even necessary, to say, write, and publish degradations. Take, for example, this quote by Julie Burchill: 'When the sex war is won prostitutes should be shot as collaborators for their terrible betrayal of all women.' How's that for a way to support women.

Slut shaming of this kind is at least as old as *Notorious*, with Ingrid Bergman's slinky outfits, drinking problem, and reckless driving. Levy's right, that women are betraying other women, but I think she's got it the wrong way round. It's the feminists who have taken up the finger-wagging role of the patriarchy.

So, yeah. I turned in my metaphorical feminism membership card because you know what? It sucks to have people write national newspaper columns about how much they not only hate people like you, but also you in particular. It's disappointing to find the much-lauded feminist writings of your day have all the depth and insight of a *Heat* article.

A lot of feminists go around clutching their pearls at the thought that there are women like me who don't want to be among their ranks. A lot of them also spend considerable effort delineating exactly who is a 'real' woman or an 'authentic' feminist and good enough to be on their team. Often, the same people are doing both of these things. It doesn't take a genius to point out the irony.

How, for instance, does it benefit feminism to ridicule people like Jordan? You might not like her body of work (so to speak), and be mystified by her success, but it's not like she was going to be the next Nobel prizewinner in physics anyway. She uses her abilities to the utmost, and she is famous neither for whose daughter she is nor whose wife she is. Bootstraps and pluck, nothing more and nothing less. That is still a strikingly uncommon distinction in this country, even today.

Jordan is to a lot of people what Madonna is to the middlebrow chattering classes: a woman whose razor-sharp business acumen has trumped her modest artistic talents. Well, I say good for her. And it's a shame so many rush to write her off, and other women like her, because they like pink clothes and don't talk posh.

This tendency for the critics and commentators to draw a line between women who 'respect themselves' and anyone who has ever waxed their pubes, is based on a failure to acknowledge the ways in which an entity can differ from itself. It is not acceptable to accuse a woman of being inauthentic simply because her choices differ from the ones you might make. A stripper is a woman. We are women. The category is big enough to handle us all, from born women to trans-women to those who simply question their gender and sexuality. It is strong enough to handle all women's histories, be they Ivy League-educated, Page Three models, or living on the streets.

The intolerant narrative in which women who display sexuality are victims and must be educated or otherwise made to pay, and in which men are portrayed as stupid or uncontrollable predators, is a trope common in many forms. It also raises its ugly, judgemental head in everything from fundamentalist propaganda to horror films. It seems women, regardless of the gaze – be it male or female – are inevitably ruined by raucous behaviour. There's a judgement suitable to every point of the ideological spectrum: they have sinned, gone wild, been tricked, or internalised the oppressor. Take your pick.

People like me are far from the first to be turned off by a movement that trivialises and rejects our concerns. Feminism has a long and storied history of excluding people it should be embracing as allies –

sex workers, transwomen, women of colour, to name just a few. The message seems to be that feminism is so embattled, the struggle so hard, that they only have the time to really care about middle-class able-bodied Western white women right now. But that the rest of us should hold the line for our so-called sisters, who more often than not are the cruellest and most spiteful haters of all.

By and large, in the West, women are not ignorant of feminism. They are all too aware that its loudest proponents can often seem the most insecure, rejecting more women than they accept. Surely that's not very feminist. Surely that's not the point.

And whether you choose to call yourself a feminist is nowhere near as important as the life you live. To be a hardworking and determined person, to be someone who refuses to be shamed by either the left or right, is far more important to me than any philosophy. Life is not about the labels we choose. Life is about how we live it.

No one would argue that the issues surrounding sex, sex work, sexuality, and so on aren't important. And, in some cases, they are certainly the kind of things government might reasonably be concerned about. So, how to stop the cycle of Agenda Setting, Constellation Making, and Evangelising? Here are some suggestions:

Beware of policies being sold to government, not to communities.

Take, for instance, the 'sexualisation' agenda. This has largely bypassed the people whose interest is arguably the greatest (families) and gone straight to top-level consultation instead. It's not only that national government might not understand the issues at stake; they often have misaligned agendas. Solving a problem is not remotely as valuable to them as making the right noises to win votes. The kudos for bringing in a new policy can be irresistible. And if it all goes wrong, as it often does, the government can either move on to the next new policy, or can blame others for its failure.

Ask if the fundamental issues are addressed.

Almost all approaches to sex work fail to consider the diversity of factors that drive the industry. The 'Swedish model' with regard to sex work is an excellent example of this. Lots of hype, not a lot of data on whether paid sex work has actually stopped or whether anyone's life outcome has been improved as a result. One common ploy of Evangelisers is paper churn, and this helps to hide the lack of hard data. Watch the coverage of the issue and you'll eventually see proponents of the Swedish approach mention how 'pressure' is ramping up on this topic – pressure that they themselves have generated through column inches. As if this means anything other than that there are lots of people willing to believe the hype. Yes, a good idea will generate lots of coverage. So does a bad one.

Ask what qualifies these people to have more influence than you do.

The people influencing (and in some cases outright dictating) policy are often no more qualified than anyone else. And when experts are consulted, they are often tied up in industry or ideology to the point of not being able to give an unbiased assessment. The people making recommendations about the internet aren't technologically savvy, the people influencing sex education are not educators, and so on. We can, and should, demand better than that when their decisions affect our lives.

Ask if more is actually better.

There is an impression when it comes to public policy that any idea, no matter how flimsy, must be rolled out *big* and *now*. More consultations, more policies, bigger conferences, more media coverage. The 'sex trafficking' issue is a striking example of this. Few ask if the increase in activity is actually producing results – or even if the problem exists at all. I find this curious because there are ways to answer these questions. Yet I've never heard of them being used in advance of money being allocated. A good rule of thumb ought to be that more is seldom better unless there has been a sea change in the way a perceived problem is approached.

When in doubt, believe the results, not the agenda.

A rule to live by, and one for policy makers specifically. If someone claims they have a great new approach to ... well, anything ... wait for their initial results before investing heavily in their 'grand plan'. It's not hard to do – testing concepts on the small scale before conducting large experiments is a common approach in science. However, the nature of politics (and perhaps politics in the modern age) seems to heavily reward grandiose schemes and overhyped sound bites ... which takes us right back to the first point on this list.

And of course ... **When in doubt, follow the money.**

The vast majority of people influenced by Agenda Setters, Constellation Makers, and Evangelisers are not bad people. They may ignore rafts of evidence simply because it's contrary to their beliefs. They may rely on gut feelings because looking outside our own direct experience is a difficult thing to do. It's misguided feelings, not avarice, that muddy many of the issues surrounding sex. The confusion also leaves their ideals open to being hijacked and their words free for the service of aims they would probably not agree with.

Reasonable people can always be shown proof that will change their minds. I myself have been subject to a mind change or two in my time. And this is what gives me hope that eventually the idea of evidence-based policy will become reality, not just a fashionable buzzword deployed in the service of worrying agendas.

Sometimes it seems as if the media are obsessed with promoting a general view of recent changes previously derided as 'Victorian'. There are indeed parallels. The end of the nineteenth century and start of the twentieth brought new technologies to add to the dissemination of ideas through mass media (much like the internet today) ... with the predictable horror and blame that brought then, just like now. The political class made some unexpected alliances as a result; again, we see this happening. One has only to look at the upcoming US elections and some of the changes being suggested by the current UK government to see coalitions of conservative Christians and middle-class 'progressives' joining forces when it comes to general disapproval of technology and sexuality. Back then such groups used rhetoric and political influence to bring us such advancements as temperance, Prohibition, and so forth. Now there's endless 'debate' and frothing about the problem of young women going out in short skirts and having an alcopop.

It was only the immediate problems of worldwide economic depression and two devastating wars that broke this obsession with public morality. The generations that had grown up under the policies influenced by late Victorian thinking rejected them. Perhaps they did so because all of the moralising in the world could not and demonstrably did not stop true suffering and true evil from flourishing in arenas that had nothing to do with private sexuality.

Is there scope for the pendulum to swing back now, short of anticipating a global political apocalypse? There is. Information is the great leveller, always. I personally am more hopeful than pessimistic. With mainstream media becoming more aware and sceptical of the misuse of data and statistics by hugely biased interests, it's possible to foresee a time when arguing over, say, whether sex workers should be added to the sex offender's register is consigned to the minority interest of extremist groups, much like opposition to same-sex marriage is now. It is with that hope and in that spirit that I imagine a world in which reason and experience finally trump the playground demons of rumour and fear.

Acknowledgements

This book would not have been possible without the work of a large number of people in sexuality studies, sex education, and biology research. The excellent work by Belinda Brooks-Gordon, Petra Boynton, Teela Sanders, and Laura Agustín has been particularly helpful, as have other contributions by too many to list (but hopefully thoroughly credited in the endnotes!). Thanks to the Centre for Sex Work Research and Policy UK mailing list, and in particular to Michael Goodyear, for support. Commentary on current issues in sex and relationships education from Justin Hancock and Sarah Thomasin was also very useful.

I have been fortunate to get help on collecting data and finding information from loads of people. In particular I would like to thank Wendy Lyon, Anna Arrowsmith, Jane Fae Ozimek, and Catherine Stephens. Alex Zhavoronkov is the creator of the useful Funding Trends website. Shout-outs to Madison Young and Maxine Holloway for a place to crash and an excellent library to plunder. Special thanks to Furrygirl, whose writing on the leaked diplomatic cables proved invaluable.

Thank you to the team who have supported this project at every stage, from Patrick Walsh and Michael Burton, to Genevieve Pegg and all the other fantastic people at Orion – Jon, Sophie, and many, many others.

Finally, I would like to thank my superhero of a husband, who has been the first reader of this work and a worthy foil in our debates on the topics involved.

Endnotes

1. http://faculty.wcas.northwestern.edu/JMichael-Bailey/research.html

2. M Chivers, G Rieger, E Latty, JM Bailey, 'A sex difference in the specificity of sexual arousal', *Psychological Science*, 2004, 15(11): 736–44

3. AP Anokhin, S Golosheykin, E Sirevaag, S Kristjansson, JW Rohrbaugh, AC Heath, 'Rapid discrimination of visual scene content in the human brain', *Brain Research*, doi:10.1016/j.brainres.2006.03.108

4. Meredith L Chivers, Michael C Seto, Ray Blanchard, 'Gender and sexual orientation differences in sexual response to sexual activities versus gender of actors in sexual films', *Journal of Personality and Social Psychology*, December 2007, 93(6): 1108–21

5. 'Slim figure for Summers', *Edinburgh Evening News*, 22 August 2007

6. Jerry Ropelato, 'Internet pornography statistics', available at: http://internet-filter-review.toptenreviews.com/internet-pornography-statistics.html

7. A Lykins, M Meana, G Kambe, 'Detection of differential viewing patterns to erotic and non-erotic stimuli using eye-tracking methodology', *Archives of Sexual Behavior*, 2006, 35: 569–75

8. HA Rupp, K Wallen, 'Sex differences in viewing sexual stimuli: an eye-tracking study in men and women', *Hormones and Behavior*, April 2007, 51(4), 524–33

9. EO Laumann, A Paik, RC Rosen, 'Sexual dysfunction in the United States: prevalence and predictors', *Journal of the American Medical Association*, 1999, 281: 537–54

10. R Moynihan, 'The making of a disease: female sexual dysfunction', *British Medical Journal*, 2003, 326: 45

11. Liz Canner (director), *Orgasm Inc.*, documentary film, 2009

12. R Moynihan, B Mintzer, *Sex, Lies, and Pharmaceuticals: How Drug Companies Plan to Profit from Female Sexual Dysfunction*, Greystone Books, 2010

13. M King, V Holt, I Nazareth, 'Women's views of their sexual difficulties: agreement and disagreement with clinical diagnoses', *Archives of Sexual Behavior*, 2007, 36(2): 281–8

14. K Oberg, AR Fugl-Meyer, KS Fugl-Meyer, 'On categorization and quantification of women's sexual dysfunctions: an epidemiological approach', *International Journal of Impotence Research*, 2004, 16: 261–9

15. I Nazareth, P Boynton, M King, 'Problems with sexual function in people attending London general practitioners: cross-sectional study', *BMJ*, 2003, 327: 423

16. L Cosgrove et al., 'Financial ties between DSM-IV panel members and the pharmaceutical industry', *Psychotherapy and Psychosomatics*, 2006, 75: 154–60

17. R Balon, A Clayton, 'Issues for DSM-V: sexual dysfunction, disorder, or variation along normal distribution: toward rethinking DSM criteria of sexual dysfunctions', *American Journal of Psychiatry*, February 2007, 164: 198–200

18. J Lenzer, 'Boehringer Ingelheim withdraws libido drug for women', *BMJ*, 2010, 341: e570

19. W Masters, V Johnson, *Human Sexual Inadequacy*, Little, Brown & Co, Boston, 1970

20. R Basson, LA Brotto, 'Sexual psychophysiology and effects of sildenafil citrate in oestrogenised women with acquired genital arousal disorder and impaired orgasm: a randomised controlled trial', *British Journal of Obstetrics and Gynaecology*, November 2003, 110(11): 1014–24

21. Vintage, 2001

22. University of Chicago Press, 1995

23. AR Parish, 'Sex and food control in the "uncommon chimpanzee": how bonobo females overcome a phylogenetic legacy of male dominance', *Ethology and Sociobiology*, May 1994, 15(3): 157–79

24. Vanessa Woods, *Bonobo Handshake*, Gotham, New York, 2010

25. EO Laumann, JH Gagnon, RT Michael, S Michaels, *The Social Organization of Sexuality: Sexual Practices in the United States*, University of Chicago Press, Chicago, 1994

26. RC Savin-Williams, LM Diamond, 'Sexual identity trajectories among sexual-minority youths: gender comparisons', *Archives of Sexual Behavior*, 2000, 29: 607–27

27. LM Diamond, 'Sexual identity, attractions, and behavior among young

sexual-minority women over a 2-year period', *Developmental Psychology*, 2000, 36: 241–50

28. Kira Cochrane, 'Why it's never too late to be a lesbian', *Guardian*, 22 July 2010

29. B Mustanski, ML Chivers, JM Bailey, 'A review and critique of the evidence for a biological basis of human sexual orientation', *Annual Review of Sex Research*, 2002, 13: 89–140

30. Kira Cochrane, ibid.

31. Drs Hor and Sprague, 'Case of nymphomania', *Boston Medical and Surgical Journal*, 1841, 25

32. ICD-10, Code F52.7

33. A Frances, 'Normality is an endangered species: psychiatric fads and overdiagnosis', *Psychiatric Times*, 6 July 2010

34. L Payer, *Disease-Mongers: How Doctors, Drug Companies, and Insurers Are Making You Feel Sick*, Wiley & Sons, New York, 1992

35. P Carnes, *Don't Call It Love: Recovery from Sexual Addiction*, Bantam Books, New York, 1991

36. CW Black, *CNS Spectrums*, January 2000, 5(1): 26–72

37. C Groneman, 'Nymphomania: the historical construction of female sexuality', *Journal of Women in Culture and Society*, 19(2): 337–67

38. S Peele, (1985) The Meaning of Addiction: Compulsive Experience and Its Interpretation. Lexington: Lexington Books.

39. Ashley Fantz, 'Can the Christian crusade against pornography bear fruit?', CNN.com, 21 August 2011

40. S Adams, Telegraph.co.uk, 26 October 2010

41. BBC.co.uk, 26 October 2010

42. J Mercurio, 'JFK, Russell Brand, and the myth of sex addiction', *The Times*, 16 April 2009

43. TM DeFrank, *Write It When I'm Gone: Remarkable Off-the-Record Conversations with Gerald R. Ford*, GP Putnam's Sons, 2007

44. L Miller, 'Is Clinton a sex addict?' Salon.com, 26 January 1998

45. MP Levine, RR Troiden, 'The myth of sexual compulsivity', *Journal of Sex Research*, 1988, 25: 347–63

46. L Aksglaede, K Sorensen, JH Petersen, NE Skakkebaek, A Juul, 'Recent decline in age at breast development: the Copenhagen Puberty Study', *Pediatrics*, 2009, 123: e932–9

47. American Psychological Association, *Report of the APA Task Force on the*

Sexualization of Girls, APA, Washington, DC, 2007

48. Australian Senate, *Inquiry into the Sexualisation of Children in the Contemporary Media Environment,* available at: http://www.aph.gov.au/Senate/committee/eca_ctte/sexualisation_of_children/tor.htm, 2007

49. http://www.slightlyrightofcentre.com/2011/10/industry-sources-isp-porn-filter-plans.html

50. NM Malamuth, T Addison, M Koss, 'Pornography and sexual aggression: are there reliable effects and can we understand them?', *Annual Review of Sex Research,* 2000, 11: 26–91

51. C Shipman, C Kazdin. 'Teens: oral sex and casual prostitution no biggie', ABCnews.go.com, 28 May 2009

52. Wellings et al., 'Sexual behaviour in context: a global perspective', *The Lancet,* 2006, 368(9548): 1706–28

53. Wellings et al., 'Sexual behaviour in Britain: early heterosexual experience', *The Lancet,* 2001, 358(9296): 1843–50

54. Centers for Disease Control, 'United States all years: percentage of students who ever had sexual intercourse (2007)', available at: http://apps.nccd.cdc.gov/yrbss/QuestYearTable.asp?path=byHT&ByVar=CI&cat=4&quest=Q58&year=Trend&loc=XX. Accessed May 2010.

55. London School of Hygiene and Tropical Medicine, 'First global analysis of sexual behaviour', press release, 30 October 2006

56. Carmine Sarracino, Kevin Scott, Beacon Press, Boston, 2008

57. Liz Jones, 'How pop became porn', *Daily Mail,* 1 March 2010

58. Nigel Morris, 'MP: teach girls virtues of virginity', *Independent,* 5 May 2011

59. R Nixon, 'Statement about the report of the Commission on Obscenity and Pornography', 24 October 1970, archived at: http://www.presidency.ucsb.edu/ws/index.php?pid=2759

60. I Eden, *Lilith Report: Lap Dancing and Strip-Tease in the Borough of Camden,* 2003, available at: http://www.childtrafficking.com/Docs/poppy_03_lap_dancing_0109.pdf> Accessed 28 December 2010.

61. 'Corrections and clarifications', *Guardian,* January 2009, available at: http://www.guardian.co.uk/theguardian/2009/jan/12/corrections

62. R Bell, 'I was seen as an object, not a person', *Guardian,* 19 March 2008

63. T Hunt, 'Betting shops and strip clubs stand as monuments to New Labour morality', *Guardian,* 2009, available at: http://www.guardian.co.uk/commentisfree/2009/aug/06/labour-moral-market-gambling-society> Accessed 28 December 2010.

64. 'Sex assaults down since lap dance clubs opened', *Newquay Voice*, 3 March 2010, available at: http://www.newquayvoice.co.uk/news/5/article/2950/

65. P Bryant, D Linz, B Shafer, 'Government regulation of adult businesses through zoning and anti-nudity ordinances: debunking the legal myth of negative secondary effects', *Communication Law and Policy*, 2001, 6(2): 355–91

66. JL Hanna, 'Exotic dance adult entertainment: a guide for planners and policy makers', *Journal of Planning Literature*, 2005, 20(2): 116–34

67. GY Lim, ME Roloff, 'Attributing sexual consent', *Journal of Applied Communication Research*, 1999, 27(1): 1–13

68. 'Porn insiders say murder case stinks on many levels', AOL News, 9 June 2010, available at: http://www.aolnews.com/weird-news/article/porn-insiders-say-stephen-hill-murder-case-stinks/19508444

69. Alan McKee, 'The objectification of women in mainstream porn videos in Australia', *Journal of Sex Research*, 2005, 42(4): 277–90

70. E Monk-Turner, HC Purcell, 'Sexual violence in pornography: how prevalent is it?', *Gender Issues*, 1999, 17(2)

71. G Dines, B Jensen, A Russo, *Pornography: The Production and Consumption of Inequality*, Routledge, Oxford, 1997

72. Beacon Press, 2010

73. Jameson Berkow, 'Porn to get .xxx domain', *Financial Post*, 25 June 2010

74. Tony Comstock, 'Is that a boiled frog in your pocket? Or are you just happy to see me?', *Atlantic*, 12 February 2011

75. Catharine A MacKinnon, 'Pornography as defamation and discrimination', *Boston University Law Review*, 1991, 71(793)

76. Shira Tarrant, 'Porn: pleasure or profit?', *Ms Magazine*, 29 June 2010

77. E Lombardi, 'Public health and trans-people: barriers to care and strategies to improve treatment' in IH Meyer, ME Northbridge (eds), *The Health of Sexual Minorities*, Springer, 2007, 638–52

78. J Keatley, J Sevelius, 'Transgender Epidemiology', presentation, University of California San Francisco Center of Excellence for Transgender HIV Prevention, available at: http://www.slideshare.net/FrancoisFilletteBerdougo/transgender-epidemiology

79. Louis A Zurcher et al., 'The antipornography campaign: a symbolic crusade', *Social Problems*, 1971, 19(2): 217–38

80. Natasha Vargas-Cooper, 'Hard core', *Atlantic*, January/February 2011

81. 23 November 2010, available at: http://www.theyworkforyou.com/debates/?id=2010-11-23c.235.0

82. Eleanor Mills, 'OMG: porn in cyberspace', *Sunday Times*, 19 December 2010

83. ML Ybarra, KJ Mitchell, M Hamburger, M Diener-West, P Leaf, 'X-rated material and perpetration of sexually aggressive behavior among children and adolescents: is there a link?', *Aggressive Behavior*, 2011, 37(1): 863–74

84. Harris Interactive Market Research, *Growing Up With Media Wave 1 Online Methodology Report*, 2006

85. Summary articles, survey results, and additional material available at: http://www.psychologies.co.uk/put-porn-in-its-place/

86. Available at: http://www.socialcostsofpornography.org/

87. Melinda Wenner Mover, 'The sunny side of smut', *Scientific American Mind*, 22 July 2011

88. Aleksandar Štulhofer, Vesna Buško, Ivan Landripet, 'Pornography, sexual socialization, and satisfaction among young men', *Archives of Sexual Behavior*, February 2010, 39(1): 168–78

89. Alan McKee, 'The relationship between attitudes towards women, consumption of pornography, and other demographic variables in a survey of 1023 consumers of pornography', *International Journal of Sexual Health*, 2007, 19(1): 31–45

90. 'Are the effects of pornography negligible?', December 2009, available at: http://www.eurekalert.org/pub_releases/2009-12/uom-ate120109.php 01

91. TD Kendall, 'Pornography, rape, and the internet', working manuscript, July 2007, available at: http://www.toddkendall.net/internetcrime.pdf

92. Anthony D'Amato, 'Porn up, rape down', available at: *anthonydamato.law.northwestern.edu/Adobefiles/porn.pdf*

93. G Dahl, S DellaVigna, 'Does movie violence increase violent crime?', *Quarterly Journal of Economics*, 2009, 124(2): 677–734

94. R Green, *Sexual Science and the Law*, Harvard University Press, 1992

95. Article 8, March 1998, available at: http://www.sexed.org/archive/article08.html

96. 'Men and porn', 8 November 2003

97. Rimm, *Georgetown Law Journal*, June 1995, 83: 1849–934

98. 'How *Time* magazine promoted a cyberhoax', 19 July 1995, available at:

http://www.fair.org/media-beat/950719.html

99. Altered image in question available at: http://www.dailymail.co.uk/ news/article-1384529/Psychologists-warn-casual-link-internet-porn-rise-sex-offences.html

100. Denis MacShane, 'Tackling the trafficking myths', *Guardian*, 16 November 2009

101. Kalyaan, *Evidence to HAC, HC 23-II, Sixth Report on Human Trafficking in the UK*

102. July 1885, available at: http://www.attackingthedevil.co.uk/pmg/ tribute/index.php

103. H Kinnell, 'Sex workers in England and Wales: briefing paper for Department of Health, National Sexual Health Strategy', EUROPAP-UK, December 1999

104. L Cusick, H Kinnell, B Brooks-Gordon, R Campbell, 'Wild guesses and conflated meanings: estimating the size of the sex worker population in Britain', *Journal of Critical Social Policy*, 2009, 29(4): 703–19

105. S Dickson, *Sex in the City*, Eaves, 2004, available at: http:// charlottegore.s3.amazonaws.com/media/DicksonSexinCotyPoppy07.pdf

106. http://www2.ohchr.org/english/law/protocoltraffic.htm

107. Julie Bindel, 'Penalising the punters', *Guardian G2*, 21 November 2008

108. *Trafficking in Persons Report*, Office to Monitor and Combat Trafficking in Persons, US Department of State, 4 June 2008

109. 'Have sex traffic levels been exaggerated?', *Newsnight*, 21 October 2009, available at: http://news.bbc.co.uk/1/hi/programmes/newsnight/8318629. stm

110. J Edwards, D Boffey, '25,000 Ex-Slaves on the Streets of Britain', *Daily Mirror*, 19 October 2005

111. Nick Davies, 'Prostitution and trafficking: the anatomy of a moral panic', *Guardian*, 20 October 2009

112. Nick Davies, 'Inquiry fails to find single trafficker who forced anybody into prostitution', *Guardian*, 20 October 2009

113. S Shuster, 'Prostitution: Ukraine's unstoppable export', *Time*, 9 October 2010

114. Wikileaks, http://www.cablegatesearch.net/cable. php?id=06YEREVAN1019

115. Tara Conlan, Carmiola Ionescu, 'Monica's story: rescued victim of child traffickers or kidnapped by ITN crew?' *Guardian*, 23 February 2008

116. 'United Kingdom Pentameter 2 statistics of victims recovered and suspects arrested during the operational phase', United Kingdom Human Trafficking Centre, available at: http://www.soca.gov.uk/about-soca/library/doc.../122-uk-pentameter-2-statistics

117. *More or Less*, BBC Radio 4, 9 January 2009

118. Tom Whitehead, 'Two in three rescued women have vanished again', *Daily Telegraph*, 16 September 2009

119. Northern Ireland Department of Justice (DoJ), 'A strategy to manage women offenders and those vulnerable to offending behaviour 2010–2013'

120. http://www.publications.parliament.uk/pa/jt200506/jtselect/jtrights/245/24508.htm

121. BBC Radio 4, ibid.

122. Available at: www.acpo.police.uk/.../Setting%20the%20Record%20(Project%20ACUMEN)%20Aug%202010.pdf

123. R Edwards, 'Up to 12,000 foreign "sex slaves" work in British brothels', *Telegraph*, 18 August 2010

124. Available at: www.soca.gov.uk/about-soca/library/doc_download/184-nrm-annual-data-april-2009-to-march-2010

125. 'People trafficking prosecution failure "startling"', BBC.co.uk, 4 May 2010

126. Catherine Bennett, 'No trafficking? Well, there's a hell of a lot of women suffering', *Observer on Sunday*, 25 October 2009

127. Nikole Hannah-Jones, 'Analysis: despite reputation, no proof Portland is a hub for child sex trafficking', *Oregonian*, 13 January 2011

128. RJ Estes and NA Weiner, 'The commercial sexual exploitation of children in the US, Canada, and Mexico', University of Pennsylvania School of Social Work Center for the Study of Youth Policy, 19 September 2001

129. US Bureau of Justice, *Human Trafficking/Trafficking in Persons*, available at: http://bjs.ojp.usdoj.gov/index.cfm?ty=tp&tid=40

130. Bureau of Justice Statistics, Office of Justice Programs, US Department of Justice press release, 15 January 2009

131. Melissa Ditmore, *The Use of Raids to Fight Trafficking in Persons*, Sex Workers Project, 2009, available at: http://sexworkersproject.org/publications/reports/raids-and-trafficking

132. House of Commons Hansard debates, 19 January 2009, available at: http://www.parliament.the-stationery-office.co.uk/pa/cm200809/cmhansrd/cm090119/debtext/90119-0014.htm

133. *News of the World*, 1 August 2010

134. D Taylor, 'Sex workers "named and shamed" on Met Police website, *Guardian*, 6 August 2010

135. *Wrong Kind of Victim? Full Report*, the Anti-Trafficking Monitoring Group, June 2010, available at: http://www.antislavery.org/english/what_ we_do/programme_and_advocacy_work/anti_trafficking_monitoring_ group.aspx

136. 'Caught between the tiger and the crocodile', available at: http://blip.tv/ file/1159149

137. Christopher Shay, Mom Kunthear, 'Study slams trafficking law', *Phnom Penh Post*, 23 July 2009

138. Robert Carmichael, 'Cambodia cracks down on the sex industry', *Deutsche Welle*, 5 April 2010

139. 'Off the streets: arbitrary detention and other abuses against sex workers in Cambodia', Human Rights Watch, July 2010

140. Wikileaks, http://www.cablegatesearch.net/cable. php?id=06PHNOMPENH1607

141. Laura Agustín, 'Leaving home for sex: prostitution, sex work, travel, trafficking', available at: http://www.lauraagustin.com/leaving-home-for-sex

142. Ruth Rosen, *The Lost Sisterhood: Prostitution in America, 1900–1918*, the Johns Hopkins University Press, paperback edition, 1983

143. Thaddeus Russell, *A Renegade History of the United States*, Free Press/ Simon & Schuster, 2010

144. GM Blackburn, SL Ricards, 'The prostitutes and gamblers of Virginia City, Nevada 1870', *Pacific Historical Review*, 1979, 48: 239–58

145. TJ Gilfoyle, *City of Eros: New York City, Prostitution, and the Commercialization of Sex, 1790–1920*, WW Norton, 1994

146. Paula Petrik, 'Capitalists with rooms: prostitution in Helena, Montana, 1865–1900', *Montana: The Magazine of Western History*, spring 1981, 31: 33–45

147. http://webarchive.nationalarchives.gov.uk/+/http://www.homeoffice. gov.uk/crime-victims/reducing-crime/prostitution/

148. Cleis Press, 2003

149. L Agustín, 'Introduction to the cultural study of commercial sex', *Sexualities*, 2007, 10: 403

150. Suzanne Jenkins, *Beyond Gender: An Examination of Exploitation in Sex Work*, 2009

151. http://www.guardian.co.uk/education/2010/sep/07/education-graduation-oecd-university

152. http://www.poverty.org.uk/59/index.shtml

153. British Crime Survey, 2003/2004

154. C Benson, R Matthews, 'Street prostitution: ten facts in search of a policy', *International Journal of Sociology of the Law*, 1995, 23: 395–415

155. M Hester, N Westmarland, *Tackling Street Prostitution: Towards a Holistic Approach*, London, 2004

156. Ronald Weitzer, 'New directions in research on prostitution', *Crime, Law, and Social Change*, 2005, 43: 211–35

157. AL Daalder, *Lifting the Ban on Brothels: Prostitution in 2000–2001*, Netherlands Ministry of Justice, 2004

158. *John F. Decker, Prostitution: Regulation and Control*, Publications of Criminal Law Education and Research Center, New York University, 13

159. C *Woodward et al., Selling Sex in Queensland 2003: A Study of Prostitution in Queensland, Prostitution* Licensing Authority, *2004*

160. Phil Hubbard, 'Cleansing the metropolis: sex work and the politics of zero tolerance', *Urban Studies*, 2004, 41: 1687–702

161. *The Challenge of Change: A Study of Canada's Criminal Prostitution Laws*, Communication Canada, Ottawa, 2006

162. Roger Matthews, Home Office Police Research Group, 1993

163. T Sanders, 'The risks of street prostitution: punters, police, and protesters', *Urban Studies*, 2004, 41: 1703–17

164. K Pease, 'Crime reduction 2003' in M Maguire, R Morgan, R Reiner (eds), *The Oxford Handbook of Criminology*, Oxford University Press, Oxford, 948–79

165. M Horne, 'Safety tips texted to prostitutes after tolerance zone ends', *Scotsman*, 8 June 2008

166. K Keane, 'Prostitution "forced into city"', 18 November 2008, available at: http://news.bbc.co.uk/1/hi/scotland/7734480.stm

167. EW Hickey, *Serial Murderers and Their Victims*, fifth edition, Wadsworth Cengage Learning, 2010, p25

168. http://www.conference-board.org/utilities/pressDetail.cfm?press_ID=3075

169. L Clark, 'Four in ten new teachers quit over red tape and unruly pupils', *Daily Mail*, 10 July 2008

170. M Farley, A Cotton, J Lynne, S Zumbeck, F Spiwak, ME Reyes, D

Alvarez, U Sezgin, 'Prostitution and trafficking in nine countries: an update on violence and posttraumatic stress disorder', *Journal of Trauma Practice*, 2003, 2(3): 33–74

171. B Brooks-Gordon, 'Memorandum of evidence on the Criminal Justice and Immigration Bill', British Psychological Society, 2008

172. Full text of the complaint available at: http://deepthroated.files.wordpress.com/2011/09/complainttoapa_melissafarley.pdf

173. Pamela Stephenson, Julie Bindel, 'Prostitution: sex, lies and exploitation', *Guardian*, 25 September 2009

174. Julie Bindel, 'The price of a holiday fling', *Guardian*, 5 July 2003

175. Grace Hammond, 'Why money has stripped away class barriers in the sex industry', *Yorkshire Post*, 20 September 2010

176. J Jordan, 'Of whalers, diggers and "soiled doves": a history of the sex industry in New Zealand' in G Abel, L Fitzgerald, C Healy, A Taylor (eds), *Taking the Crime Out of Sex Work: New Zealand Sex Workers' Fight for Decriminalisation*, Policy Press, 2010

177. 'Big increase of sex workers a myth: latest research', Christchurch School of Medicine and Health Sciences, 2006

178. *Report of the Prostitution Law Review Committee on the Operation of the Prostitution Reform Act 2003*, available at: http://www.justice.govt.nz/policy-and-consultation/legislation/prostitution-law-review-committee/publications/plrc-report/report-of-the-prostitution-law-review-committee-on-the-operation-of-the-prostitution-reform-act-2003

179. Melissa Farley, 'What really happened in New Zealand after prostitution was decriminalized in 2003?', available at: www.prostitutionresearch.com/Report on NZ 10-29-2008.pdf

180. G Abel, L Fitzgerald, C Healy, A Taylor (eds), *Taking the Crime Out of Sex Work: New Zealand Sex Workers' Fight for Decriminalisation*, Policy Press, 2010

181. Laura Agustín, 'Big claims, little evidence: Sweden's law against buying sex', *Local*, 23 July 2010, available at: http://www.lauraagustin.com/ban-on-purchase-of-sex-helps-prevent-and-combat-prostitution-says-swedish-evaluation

182. Bedford vs Canada ruling, full document available at: *www.cbc.ca/news/pdf/bedford-ruling.pdf*

183. Robert Bork, 'Neutral principles and some First Amendment problems', *Indiana Law Journal*, 1971, 47

184. Les Horton, *Gulf Daily News*, 10 October 2010

185. Andrew Gant, *Daytona Beach News-Journal*, 15 September 2010

186. Katie Dawson, BBC News, 7 June 2010

187. Multiple sources, including:

J Ballesteros et al., 'Low seroincidence and decrease in seroprevalence of HIV among female prostitutes in Madrid', *AIDS*, 1999, 13: 1143

R Mak, J Plum, L Van Renterghem, 'Human immunodeficiency virus (HIV) infection, sexually transmitted diseases and HIV-antibody testing practices in Belgian prostitutes', *Genitourinary Medicine*, 1990; 66: 337–41

S Day, H Ward, 'Sex workers and the control of sexually transmitted disease', *Genitourinary Medicine*, 1997, 73: 161–8

R Mak (ed.), *EUROPAP: European Intervention Projects AIDS Prevention for Prostitutes*, Academia Press, Gent, 1996

J Vioque, I Hernandez-Aguado, E Garcia, et al., 'Prospective cohort study of female sex workers and the risk of HIV infection in Alicante, Spain (1986–96)', *Sexually Transmitted Infections*, 1998, 74: 284–8

M Spina, S Mancuso, A Sinicco, et al., 'Human immunodeficiency virus seroprevalence and condom use among female sex workers in Italy', *Sexually Transmitted Diseases*, 1998, 25: 451–4

188. H Ward, S Day, JN Weber, 'Risky business: health and safety in the sex industry over a 9-year period', *Sexually Transmitted Infections*, 1999, 75: 340–3

189. Multiple sources, including:

S Day, H Ward, JRW Harris, 'Prostitute women and public health', *BMJ*, 1988, 297: 1585

H Ward, S Day, J Mezzone, et al., 'Prostitution and risk of HIV: female prostitutes in London', *BMJ*, 1993, 307: 356–8

'Renewing the focus: HIV and other sexually transmitted infections in the United Kingdom in 2002', an update, Health Protection Agency, London, 2003

G Kinghorn, 'Patient access to GUM clinics', *Sexually Transmitted Infections*, 2001, 77: 1–3

H Ward, S Day, A Green, K Cooper, JN Weber, 'Declining prevalence of STI in the London sex industry, 1985 to 2002', *Sexually Transmitted Infections*, 2004, 80: 374–6

190. Dukers-Muijrers, Niekamp, Brouwers, Hoebe, 'Older and swinging: need to identify hidden and emerging risk groups at STI clinics', *Sexually*

Transmitted Infections, 2010, 86: 315–17

191. 'FPA warns of rising STIs and poor sexual health in the over 50s', press release, Family Planning Association, 14 September 2010, available at: http://www.fpa.org.uk/Pressarea/Pressreleases/2010/14September2010-2

192. Wikileaks, http://www.cablegatesearch.net/cable.php?id=06BERLIN1687

193. Wikileaks, http://www.cablegatesearch.net/cable.php?id=06FRANKFURT4232

194. C Daniels, 'World Cup "didn't fuel SA sex industry"', Digitalspy.co.uk, 23 October 2010

195. Accessed at: http://www.huntalternatives.org/download/2000_abtreport_8_10.pdf

196. https://twitter.com/#!/bindelj/status/1359241025683456

197. 'Adolescent girls in the United States sex trade tracking study results for May, 2010', the Schapiro Group, available at: http://extras.twincities.com/pdf/May2010TrackingStudy.pdf

198. 'Public's views on prostitution', Ipsos MORI survey, 4 September 2008

199. http://www.quora.com/Human-Trafficking/Why-is-it-so-common-to-include-voluntary-prostitution-in-the-category-of-sex-trafficking

200. Martin Cizmar, Ellis Conklin, Kristen Hinman, *Village Voice*, 29 June 2011

201. Joe Morris, 'Young prostitute can't sue *Village Voice*', Courthouse News Service, 19 August 2011

202. Ashton Kutcher, http://aplusk.posterous.com/why-fight-it-could-be-your-daughter-your-niec

203. http://www.publications.parliament.uk/pa/cm200809/cmhansrd/cm081218/text/81218w0034.htm

204. http://www.pentameter.police.uk/news.php?id=5

205. JE McGaha, A Evans, 'Where are the victims?' *Intercultural Human Rights Law Review*, 239

206. Pamela Engel, 'Senator asks for more scrutiny of human trafficking grants', *Scripps Howard Foundation Wire*, 16 September 2011, available at: http://www.shfwire.com/node/5996

207. http://www.guardian.co.uk/society/2011/feb/15/women-refuge-chief-protest-cuts

208. Available at: http://www.charity-commission.gov.uk/SHOWCHARITY/RegisterOfCharities/CharityWithPartB.aspx?Registered

CharityNumber=275048&SubsidiaryNumber=0

209. http://heresycorner.blogspot.com/2011/04/feminists-and-evangelicals-compete-to.html

210. http://www.guardian.co.uk/commentisfree/2009/apr/03/prostitution-humantrafficking

211. http://liberalconspiracy.org/2008/10/22/sex-work-figure-fixing-and-victorian-philanthropy/

212. http://liberalconspiracy.org/2009/10/21/new-credibility-gap-in-sex-trafficking-estimates/

213. http://www.fundingtrends.org/?keywords=trafficking%2C+%22lung+cancer%22

214. http://www.fundingtrends.org/?keywords=trafficking%2C+%22lung+cancer%22%2C+malnutrition%2C+malaria%2C+tuberculosis

215. Emi Koyama, 'Trade secrets', *Bitch* magazine, 2011, 53

216. Alice Fishburn, Hattie Garlick, 'We thought of ourselves as calendar girls', *The Times*, 14 May 2010

217. Melissa Benn, '*Living Dolls* by Natasha Walter, *The Equality Illusion* by Kat Banyard', *Independent*, 5 March 2010

218. Elissa Bassist, 'Sleep your way to a book deal', Salon.com, 8 May 2010

About the author

Dr Brooke Magnanti is a science researcher who studied genetic epidemiology at master's level and did her doctoral studies with the Dept of Forensic Pathology at the University of Sheffield. Her professional interests include population-based research, standards of evidence, and human biology and anthropology. In 2009, it was revealed that she is an ex-call girl and author of the bestselling Belle de Jour series of memoirs, which were adapted into the ITV series *Secret Diary of a Call Girl* starring Billie Piper.

Index